AN INTRODUCTION TO
ANTHROPOSOPHICAL MEDICINE

Extending the Art of Healing

Victor Bott, MD

Sophia Books

The information in this book is not intended to be taken as a replacement for medical advice. Any person with a condition requiring medical attention should consult a qualified medical practitioner or suitable therapist. The directions for treatment of particular diseases are given for the guidance of medical practitioners only, and should not be prescribed by those who do not have a medical training.

Sophia Books
Hillside House, The Square
Forest Row, RH18 5ES

www.rudolfsteinerpress.com

Published by Sophia Books 2004
An imprint of Rudolf Steiner Press

First published in English by Rudolf Steiner Press in 1978 and reprinted 1982. Translated from French by F.L. Wheaton and G. Douch. This edition has been edited, revised and updated by Matthew Barton. Originally published in French under the title *Médicine Anthroposophique, Un élargissement de l'art de guérir*, by Triades-Éditions, Paris 1972

Translation © Rudolf Steiner Press 2004

A catalogue record for this book is available from the British Library

ISBN 1 85584 177 0

Cover by Andrew Morgan Design
Typeset by DP Photosetting, Aylesbury, Bucks.
Printed and bound in Great Britain by Cromwell Press Limited, Trowbridge, Wilts.

CONTENTS

PART THREE
THE FOUR CARDINAL ORGANS

PART FOUR
SOME SPECIAL PROBLEMS

Foreword

by Dr Peter Grünewald

In the early years of the twentieth century a group of doctors and medical students asked Rudolf Steiner, an Austrian scientist and philosopher, to develop a holistic approach to illness and the art of healing that encompassed the human being's spiritual, emotional and physical existence. As a result Rudolf Steiner gave a series of lectures on illness, health and the art of healing from a spiritual and holistic perspective. Applying the methods of scientific and philosophical research to the spiritual dimension of the human being and the natural world, he collaborated with doctors to develop a system of medicine which has always regarded itself as an extension of mainstream medicine rather than an alternative. The method of diagnosis and therapy Steiner developed looks at the human being as a body, mind and spirit unity within the context of the person's social environment. It tries to help patients find a personal understanding of the *meaning of chronic illness as a vehicle for spiritual growth and personal transformation*, empowering them where possible to overcome illness or otherwise integrate illness into their life in a meaningful way.

One of the aims of treatment can be to help the patient find a stronger relationship to his/her own inner self. It can facilitate the development of new, creative personal and social skills, and—if the patient wishes—enable him/her to develop inner freedom, self-determination and a caring approach to others and to life in general. In this context the art of healing can come to support the process of individual human development, whereby partial tendencies of our personality are integrated into the wholeness of our human experience.

Together with Dr Ita Wegman, one of the physicians close to him, Rudolf Steiner wrote and published a book called *Fundamentals of Therapy: an Extension to the Art of Healing* (now published under the title of *Extending Practical Medicine*).

Dr Wegman founded a clinic for inpatients and outpatients at Arlesheim, Switzerland, where doctors and a dedicated team of therapists have continued to practise the methods of anthroposophical medicine to this day, treating patients with chronic physical illnesses. This clinic, which is close to the Goetheanum—the general headquarters of the anthroposophical movement and the 'School of Spiritual Science' in Dornach—has now developed into a teaching clinic for anthroposophical medicine.

This medical system was one of the earliest to adopt a holistic approach, and it remains one of the most comprehensive to this day. Steiner always insisted that his medical approach *should only be practised by or in cooperation with conventionally qualified doctors* since his intention was to *extend* the art of medicine rather than substitute something quite different.

Worldwide and especially in Germany, the Netherlands and Switzerland, more than a thousand general practitioners and consultants practise anthroposophical medicine. In free independent practice and in a number of hospitals and clinics, they are an integrated part of mainstream health care systems. There is also a university, Herdecke in Witten, Germany, as well as a number of teaching hospitals and training centres encompassing nearly all existing medical specialisms.

In Britain, some anthroposophical doctors work in private practice, some in the National Health Service, some in Steiner schools, and others in homes for children with special needs. There are two clinics providing anthroposophical medicine in the UK and there are many more in other parts of the world.

In Britain this type of medicine is regulated by the Anthroposophical Health Council, a self-regulatory organization for anthroposophical health professionals, which promotes education, training and quality assurance for its members.

One branch of anthroposophical medicine is devoted to therapeutic work with children and adolescents with learning or emotional and behavioural difficulties. In Britain and many other countries there is a large number of special needs residential schools. The approach adopted integrates care, education and medicine/therapy in a mutually enhancing, holistic way.

Anthroposophical medicine is a very comprehensive system, which encompasses a number of diagnostic and therapeutic methods and principles. Some of the more important ones are touched on in this book by Victor Bott.

Rudolf Steiner, in creating his system of medicine, drew on Johann Wolfgang Goethe's scientific research method. Goethe's writings on natural science are very little known, but in his studies on light, colour, botany, meteorology and human anatomy he developed a method of research that can help open a spiritual dimension in our experience of nature and the human being. Goethe's method is less an analytical than a synthetic one. Rather than immediately judging the content of our perceptions, his approach allows the objects and phenomena of nature—such as the development of a plant or the changes of the clouds of the sky—to live within the human soul and sensibility, so that the changing images produced in us in this way develop, unfold and metamorphose in time. Experiencing this waxing and waning of organic life within the human soul allows the marrying of two opposite poles of human nature: active observation and exact sensorial imagination. Goethe called this new skill and research tool *Anschauende Urteilskraft*, which very loosely translated means 'the power of intuitive judgement drawing on creative perception'. This refers, in other words, to our ability to come to insights by experiencing the content of perception in a dynamic way.

In applying this inner activity to researching organic nature one learns to experience the development of organic life in fundamental polarities, such as birth and death, waxing and waning, light and darkness, straight line and curve, etc.

Metamorphosis of organic life appears to result from a struggle between opposite form tendencies—such as straight line and curve. One can, for example, see this in the polarity between sperm and ovum or, in the plant, between upward-striving vertical tendencies (stem) and outspreading horizontal tendencies (leaf). The imaginative capacities of the human soul partake in this interplay of opposites and learn to inwardly recreate the world of natural phenomena, instead of just researching the dead products of life. This is, broadly, the difference between an understanding derived from dissection and anatomy and one which enters into the dynamic of living processes. In experiencing life as an organic development in time, nature's laws and synthesizing forces can reveal themselves in a different manner, allowing the researcher to participate inwardly in the process of creation. Applied to researching the human constitution in illness and health, this method offers the researcher insights that complement modern scientific research. The same method applied to the human mind and emotions leads us to an understanding of human soul life between the polarities of cognition (perception, concept and image formation) and activity (force, instinct, desire, drive).

This polarity between intellectual onlooker consciousness and active intuitive involvement in changing the world or satisfying our physical and emotional needs is mediated by our *feelings and emotions*. These themselves live within the polarity of *sympathy,* which embraces the world and stimulates activity, and *antipathy,* which creates an emotional distance and helps us to be awake and attentive in our cognition. (Steiner's use of these two terms is far broader and less subjectively coloured than our common understanding of them. He sees sympathy and antipathy as fundamental forces imbuing all our activity in both conscious and unconscious ways.)

Anger and fear are also a polarity within human emotions, as are the feelings of courage and devotion. One can even speak of *cold* emotions and feelings, which create distance and thus support cognition, and *warm/hot* emotions and feelings, which can lead to will activity.

Mental health is therefore the ability to keep these extreme poles within a dynamic balance. Its absence can lead to illnesses in which one pole is predominant, such as the cognition pole in symptoms of obsessive compulsive disorder, depression, phobia, anxiety disorders, autistic spectrum disorders, etc. On the other hand, the activity pole is predominant in conditions or symptoms such as ADHD, hyperactivity, mania, delusions, and uncontrolled anger with aggression and violence.

Our feelings and emotions, which are based organically on the activity of the *rhythmic system (breathing and circulation),* balance the cognition process, which is based on the activity of the *nerve-sense system (CNS),* and the will processes, which are based on the *metabolic-limb system.*

These concepts arise from an overall view in anthroposophical medicine that the human being can be regarded as having a *threefold nature,* related to the basic human functions of thinking, feeling and will. The author develops the organic aspects of human threefoldness in his second chapter 'The Human Triad' and lays herewith one of the foundations for a holistic and dynamic understanding of illness and health.

The rhythmic system, in balancing the opposite, polar functions of the other two systems described above, is inherently health-creating. It is thus evident that healing processes require a strengthening of this rhythmic system (see Chapter 3, 'Health and Disease').

Careful observation of patients with organic conditions will show that *physical illness usually goes hand-in-hand with a distinct alteration of consciousness*—such as weakness of the will and indecisiveness in acute or chronic liver disease; the swing between lethargy and over-emotionality in some forms of kidney disease; a tendency to obsessive thoughts or repetition in some forms of degenerative lung diseases; a tendency to delusions during the inflammatory and exudative phase of pulmonary tuberculosis; feelings of existential anxiety and abnormal conscience in some forms of heart disease, etc. (See Part Three, 'The Cardinal Four Organs', Chapters 10, 11, 12 and 13.) These emotional and psychological expressions of physical ailments have been well researched by writers, for example the pulmonary tuberculosis that figures in Thomas Mann's *Magic Mountain*.

At a physical level illnesses can be regarded as a disturbance of the dynamic functional balance of the three systems described above.

A predominance of the anabolic, warmth-creating and dynamic functions of the metabolic system can express itself in the tendency towards inflammatory illnesses and fever.

A predominance of the catabolic, cooling, form-creating and movement-inhibiting tendencies of the nerve-sense system can lead to degenerative 'cold' illnesses, like arteriosclerosis, cancer, lithiasis (stone-formation tendencies), constipation and other metabolic diseases, such as diabetes and gout, etc.

Some illnesses are combinations of both tendencies of inflammation and degeneration, such as in chronic rheumatism, pulmonary tuberculosis or chronic hepatitis. (See Chapter 6, 'Inflammation and Sclerosis'.)

It is the task of anthroposophical medical research to explore the relationship between nature and the human being in illness and health. The research method of Goethe outlined above is one of the central tools to do this. The work of exploring the relationship between man and nature was done prior to Rudolf Steiner by Paracelsus (Theophrastus Bombastus von Hohenheim), the famous Swiss physician and pharmacologist. He delved into ancient spiritual wisdom with a modern scientific consciousness, relating to the *connection and interrelation between nature (macrocosm) and man (microcosm)*. By applying his scientifically trained mind to this research, he obtained a number of deep insights into the relationship between certain minerals, metals or plants and human illness and consciousness. These insights led to the production of natural remedies and their application in moderating and healing patients' ailments.

Although Steiner's research is not based on Paracelsus' insights, they agree with each other in many areas. Anthroposophical medicine, like the medical system of Paracelsus, also distinguishes *a fourfold structure of the human being* (see Chapter 1, 'The Four Constituent Elements of the Human Being'). The fourfold system, as distinct from the threefold system described earlier, is as follows.

Firstly, there is the *physical body* which is filled out by the *material substances* of the natural world.

Secondly, the human being has a *'body' of life forces*, the so-called *etheric body*, which he has in common with the *plant* world. The life forces, known as etheric forces, operate through the medium of water—hence life is *dependent on water*. Life forces cannot work without it, e.g. seeds will not germinate without water. In the human being the etheric body is responsible for regeneration of the human organization, which is affected by exhausting and illness-creating stimuli from within (strong, sometimes destructive emotions, such as anger, fear, anxiety) and from without (e.g. environmental influences, poor nutrition and toxins). In sleep the regenerating activity of the etheric organization is predominant. During waking these forces are partly transformed into consciousness, such as memory, concept formation, etc. This leads to a tiring of the human organization during waking along with the need to regenerate again in sleep (see Chapter 5, 'Sleeping and Waking'). The etheric body contains formation and growth forces for the human organs. These forces are transformed into consciousness, and during early childhood become the organic base for the concept-forming process within the brain. The etheric body sustains *memory, routine and habit formation*. A flexible routine can help to recreate new life forces, which in turn sustain health.

Thirdly, the human being possesses a *'body' of soul forces* which rules, informs and structures the physical and etheric in such a way that these become capable of sensation and feeling. The human being has this third feature in common with the *animals*. In contradistinction to plants it gives them movement and the ability to experience sensations. This body is called the *astral body*, and the so-called astral forces operate as *consciousness-building* forces via the gaseous constituents of the body, i.e. the air or dissolved gases. The astral body is the carrier of emotions, drives, desires and instincts; if these are destructive or too extreme, the human organization can become exhausted and fall ill with time. To stay well, it needs the counterbalance of the etheric organization and the moderating, regulating and balancing effect of the ego, the fourth aspect of the human being (see below).

The fourth part of the human being, and the one which distinguishes us from all the other kingdoms of nature, is the *ego*. This, as we have seen, endows human beings with *indi-*

viduality. The ego holds the balance between the other forces, particularly the astral and the etheric. The medium through which ego forces can operate is *warmth*. The ego expresses itself in a number of specific human skills, such as the *ability to walk upright, to speak and to reflect,* as well as through the *ability to develop self-awareness, self-knowledge and increasing self-determination.* The ego gradually transforms the forces at work in other parts of human nature and *individualizes the influences of inheritance and of the social environment.* The ego as bearer of individuality is regarded as the *essential kernel of the human being.* Illnesses we have experienced can be transformed into skills and abilities through the activity of the ego.

Anthroposophical medicine tries to support individual development by attempting to strengthen the ego as the human being's innermost nucleus in his striving for *developing freedom (self-determination) and empathy.* It is ego-orientated—in other words, it helps the ego to balance polarities of forces and extremes, and to gradually transform human nature.

Potentized anthroposophical remedies from the three kingdoms of nature, either as single remedies or in specifically developed composition, as well as *herbal (non-potentized) remedies* can help bring about transformation of the (sick) human constitution.

A number of anthroposophical remedy compositions for specific conditions, such as the treatment of migraine, digestive disorders, liver disease, etc., as well as remedies for the treatment of mental illness, were either developed by doctors and pharmacists in cooperation with Rudolf Steiner or have been based on his research.

These anthroposophical remedies seem to stimulate and strengthen the ego in its attempt to overcome the one-sidedness of the human constitution. *Instead of suppressing symptoms they stimulate the development of new personal and human skills*. At the end of a successful treatment cycle for a chronic condition, over several weeks or months patients often remark that they not only feel better in themselves but feel much more in charge of their own life. They frequently seem able to deal with adverse life circumstances more creatively and no longer feel themselves to be victims of circumstances. Extreme thoughts, emotions and fixed pathological habits can be lifted into consciousness and, if wished, be transformed. Symptoms of physical illness can be moderated and sometimes even overcome.

In this book, Victor Bott, gives a systematic introduction to anthroposophical medicine. In Part One, he outlines the basic constituents of the human being, and shows how a *dynamic* understanding of them provides insight into the diagnosis of illness and what is the most effective therapeutic intervention. Thus, for example, he introduces elements of an understanding of the human constitution in its one-sidedness or disharmonies that lead to a predisposition to developing particular diseases. He shows how these insights aid in the understanding of the nature and treatment of insomnia, and also of inflammation and sclerosis (two polar conditions).

Part Two consists of an introduction to the development of the human being during his/her first 21 years of life. In each of the three seven-year periods, outlined in Chapters 7, 8 and 9, the young human being needs different challenges and different means of support for his/her cognitive, emotional, will and moral development. The child's consciousness is reflected in his/her parallel physical development.

A disturbing influence arising from the physical and social environment and/or from the inherited forces can either lead to the characteristic illnesses of this age group or to particular diseases later on in life. Some of these illnesses, their treatment, and also their meaning, i.e. possible beneficial effects in human development, are discussed.

Part Three introduces the four main organ systems—lung, liver, kidney and heart—as connected with the four basic constitutional elements, and shows how they underlie both physical and mental illness. Looking at the relationship between organ processes and health, and human temperament and consciousness, Dr Bott examines specific organic illnesses as well as specific mental health problems, such as schizophrenia, mania and depression.

Part Four concludes this book by introducing an extended understanding of the causes underlying constitutional factors leading to conditions like cancer, disturbances of the menstrual cycle and diseases of the skin. The implications for therapeutic interventions extending conventional approaches are outlined.

Victor Bott's book is a valuable contribution to the understanding of the principles behind anthroposophic medicine, allowing the reader to gain a deeper insight into the nature of the human being, and of illness and health from a holistic point of view.

Peter Grünewald
April 2004

INTRODUCTION

*'So that all the paths which lead to
goodness should not be closed.'*

Solzhenitsyn

The art of healing has always reflected man's ideas of his own nature. Modern medicine has thus been strongly influenced by the materialistic thought of the nineteenth century, tending to regard the human organism as a sort of test tube in which certain processes analogous to laboratory experiments take place. But the practitioner called to his patient's bedside knows that this way of looking at things is inadequate, in the face of day-to-day reality. Perhaps we can consider this as demonstrating that our scientific picture of man is incomplete. This book aims to recreate this picture and widen our conception of the human being, so as to create an art of healing more in harmony with tangible human reality—a medicine really able to encompass that reality.

This wider picture of man has already been given to us by Rudolf Steiner, the founder of anthroposophy. The practical results he obtained in spheres as diverse as agriculture, the art of education and medicine vouch for the validity of the path he pursued. Anthroposophy is a way of knowledge which can be followed with the same rigour as that of modern scientific research.

When beginning the study of anthroposophy one is struck by the link, or synthesis, it creates between disparate human disciplines. For example, is it not surprising to find a link between two fields as divergent as geology and medicine? Yet, if we consider that earth and man have evolved together, we can understand more readily why certain rocks provide a basis for a remedy for an organ which began to develop during the same epoch as that rock. We shall find other examples of this kind later.

We are all familiar with the amazing technical progress that the modern development of the intellect has brought about. But this intellectual discipline can itself sometimes hamper development of a sound knowledge of man and the universe. We find it hard to be unprejudiced in the spheres that lie outside our weighing, measuring and reckoning, for we have all become so accustomed from our school days to think in terms of physics, chemistry and mathematics. To declare that the spheres outside the reach of our physical senses simply do not exist is a dogmatic belief with as little basis as a blind belief in the opposite opinion. In his present state of consciousness Western man has estranged himself from the idea of a spiritual world because he tends to think he can only study objectively what presents itself through the senses.

Rudolf Steiner found other ways of working, and he described them in detail. Through his research in supersensible spheres he has shown, among other things, that man cannot be described as consisting of a physical body only, but that he also has a soul and a spirit. His extensive works include close on six thousand lectures which have nearly all been taken down in shorthand, and many of them published.

It would be quite beyond the scope of this book to undertake a thorough study of anthroposophy, therefore some of the ideas we put forward may seem strange or dogmatic to the uninformed reader. If he feels he would like to look more closely into this underlying body of thought, I strongly advise him to consult the works of Rudolf Steiner, many of which have been published in English. He will find some of the relevant titles mentioned in the notes and the further reading list. I shall try, nevertheless, to develop my argument gradually, so that everyone can follow.

Respect for freedom of thought is a basic tenet of anthroposophy. Rudolf Steiner said many times that he did not ask anyone to believe what he said, but asked people to test and verify it. Many of his statements have indeed been verified subsequently. For example, in a lecture he gave on 3 July 1924, speaking of lunar rocks, Steiner said that they differ from earth minerals and have a vitrified aspect. There were of course neither space rockets nor astronauts at that time. How many scientists would have ridiculed such an assertion only a short while ago! But the astronauts from Apollo 11 and 12 have brought back rocks containing small glass balls whose origin has yet to be explained. Another example of remarkably prescient insight is Steiner's statement that cattle fed a non-vegetarian diet would go mad—since proven in the BSE crisis!

I was really feeling sadly unprepared for the task of embarking on the practice of anthroposophical medicine, when I owned my misgivings to a colleague, Dr Marty of Basel, to whom I dedicate this book, and who already had long years of practice behind him. 'You must have the courage to start,' he said. I did as he said, and tried to devote as long as possible to each patient. I was surprised to find, and to develop the conviction, that there are no patients to whom anthroposophical medicine cannot bring help in one way or another.

I have written this book with the hope of sharing this conviction with those who despair at the shortcomings of present-day medical knowledge, and with the aim of giving them the rudiments they need to start on their way along this path.

Part One

MAN IN THE LIGHT OF ANTHROPOSOPHY

It is not possible to gain a full picture of the human being by considering his material aspect alone. Only by looking at him as a whole, composed of body, soul and spirit, can we arrive at a comprehensive idea of man. Of these three aspects, the body is itself divisible into two elements: the first can be measured and weighed, and is related to space, and the second makes us a living being subject to constant change, and relates us to time. There are thus four elements that together constitute the whole human being.

Considered from the aspect of his visible form and physical functions, man also shows himself to be a whole composed of two opposite polarities, united by a central harmonizing element, together forming a threefold whole.

Man is therefore at one and the same time a fourfold and a threefold being. It is only possible to understand him fully by linking together these two aspects, as anthroposophy does. We shall attempt to explain this in the first part of this book.

1

THE FOUR CONSTITUENT ELEMENTS
OF THE HUMAN BEING

When we study the mineral world's physical and chemical processes, we find a potential for decay and destruction of life but no possibility of maintaining life, still less of creating it. With the aid of heat, cold, electricity or the various chemical substances, we can kill a plant, but we cannot by those means bring a mineral to life. To attempt to understand life by applying to it ideas acquired by the study of the mineral kingdom leads to a dead end, to questions which we cannot honestly answer. While the regions formerly labelled 'terra incognita' have disappeared from our scientific atlases, the number of unanswered questions about life itself have increased. It was thought that they had been solved by theories derived from the mineral world, but one after another these have been shown to be false.

If, instead of exploring further and further into the micro-realms of the infinitely small, we attempt to study vital processes as a whole, and if we set aside prejudices which are all the stronger for being presented in a scientific guise, we rapidly reach a first conclusion—that life is always at war with, or in opposition to, the physico-chemical processes of the mineral world. We can find numerous examples of this in the vegetable kingdom. Thus, a mineral is subject to gravity and has a tendency to subside to a lower level. The plant, on the other hand, grows in opposition to these forces of gravity. The sap rises in the stem not by means of osmosis, but in spite of osmosis: by overcoming it. The dead substances of the mineral world have a tendency to liberate energy when mixed together and thus to descend to a lower level of energy. In the plant, on the contrary, the final level of energy is higher than that at the beginning. This necessarily implies the bringing into play of considerable forces. Newton arrived intuitively at the idea of gravity on seeing the apple fall, but he does not seem to have asked himself about the no less mysterious matter of how the apple reached the end of the branch. The apple which falls from the tree escapes from the laws of life and is subject only to the laws of the physical world, such as gravitation which is a force directed towards the centre of the earth. But as long as the apple is part of the apple tree, it is subject to cosmic forces, solar forces and others working in the opposite direction to gravity. These forces do not act indifferently on the substances that they borrow from the physical world. They make their choice of them, select, refine and direct them, and confer on them new properties and, in a more general manner organize them in accordance with a pre-established plan proper to each species. These forces not only affect structure and growth but also reproduction.

These forces, without which there is no life, anthroposophy calls *etheric forces* or *formative forces*. They must not be confused with the hypothetical vital force of which nineteenth-century science spoke, which was merely a fiction intended to throw a veil of modesty over that of which one was ignorant. Neither have they anything to do with the hypothetical ether of the physicists. These etheric or formative forces constitute for every living being a kind of second body, the *etheric body*, intimately united with the physical body which alone is accessible to our senses.

It would be easy to object that no one has ever seen this etheric body, to which one could reply that no one has ever seen electricity, magnetism or gravitation, forces which we know only from their effects. In the same way everyone can understand the existence of etheric forces from their effects. The objection that they are not visible is therefore no more valid than that which a colour-blind person could make to the existence of colours. But while a colour-blind person will remain so all his life, there exists in a germinal state in all of us a spiritual eye which it is possible to develop, permitting the perception of etheric forces and their description down to the smallest detail.[1]

Although the etheric forces are of a nature entirely different from electro-magnetic forces, there is a means of demonstrating them both which presents a certain similarity. You know that if one places a sheet of paper sprinkled with iron filings on top of a magnet, the iron filings arrange themselves in such a way as to form the image of the magnetic field. If we let a salt solution crystallize out after having added to it some drops of an extract from a living plant or tissue, we shall see the crystals arrange themselves to give an image of the etheric forces of the living substance studied.

It was E. Pfeiffer[2] who patiently developed this method, suggested to him by Rudolf Steiner, and gave to it the name *sensitive crystallization.* It is not a quantitative but a qualitative method. The resemblance with the method of demonstrating the magnetic field is, however, only superficial for, whereas the picture of a magnetic field always remains the same, the pictures produced by sensitive crystallization present an infinite variety. An experienced observer can tell you to what species the extract added to the salt solution belongs (in practice one generally uses copper chloride) and can even tell if it is from the root, the leaf or the flower. The pictures produced vary also according to the quality of the substance used, and one can differentiate in this way between plants cultivated by different methods. Applied to the study of human blood, this sensitive crystallization is a valuable aid in the diagnosis of diseases. It allows certain disease characteristics to be distinguished and may also indicate in which organs the disease is localized.

The etheric forces need a material support, that is to say a medium, in order to manifest themselves, and water is, in fact, always the medium for these forces. When a plant is deprived of water the etheric forces withdraw and the plant dies. They can remain dormant in the seed for years. We need only water the seed in order to see the formative forces become active once more, revealing themselves in the germination, growth and development of the plant. The substances borrowed from the mineral world are transformed and raised to the level of the vegetable kingdom. They then acquire new properties which they did not have in the mineral kingdom. From the chemical points of view there is no difference, for chemical analysis reveals only properties belonging to the mineral kingdom. Nevertheless the new properties conferred by the etheric forces can be demonstrated, provided that the appropriate methods are employed. Chemical methods appropriate to the mineral world are obviously not appropriate to this realm.

The plant has, as we have seen, become partly independent of gravity. The animal, a being living in the horizontal plane, seems to have lost this faculty. But this is only apparently so, for the animal has transformed into a dynamic property what the plant possesses in a static form. The animal can change its position, jump, climb, even fly. This capacity for movement, which distinguishes it from the plant, is inseparable from another faculty—that of feeling. Feeling may be expressed both in desire and fear. Attraction and repulsion, we could say, or *sympathy* and *antipathy*[3] are the poles between which the animal perpetually swings. These affective states are inside it and are manifested externally by movement. The inner content, which we may call soul or psyche, is the result of external stimuli having been interiorized a shorter or

longer time previously. The animal, its psyche and its movement are so closely connected that the Romans, feeling this
relationship so strongly, indicated them by words etymo-
logically closely related, which we find again as: *animal*,
animated, and the French *âme* (meaning 'soul', in Latin
anima). For only that which is animated, which possesses a
soul, can be endowed with movement proper.

Thus with the animal we are able to observe a new faculty
which we do not find in the plant, that of interiorization. In
the animal the exterior world becomes interiorized. This
shows itself in its very structure. It is sufficient to compare the
leaf, the respiratory organ of the plant, with that of the animal—the pulmonary alveolus—in order to realize this. The
leaf is surrounded by air which is outside it. In the pulmonary
alveolus the air is within, surrounded by the organ (Fig. 1),

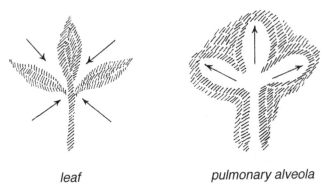

leaf   pulmonary alveola

Fig. 1

and at the same time movement appears in the process of
respiration. We even find this process of interiorization again
at a very early embryological stage. When the ovum begins to
develop it forms a ball of cells called a *morula* from its
resemblance to a small mulberry (Fig. 2). In the next stage the
cells range themselves at the periphery and form a kind of

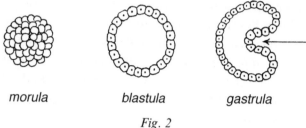

morula   blastula   gastrula

Fig. 2

little bladder called a *blastula*. From this moment one part of the wall of the blastula becomes indented and we arrive at the stage of the *gastrula*, so called because of its resemblance to a stomach. This indentation, called invagination, is a typically animal manifestation of interiorization. The plant never passes beyond the blastula stage.

We must ask ourselves what causes this gastrula formation. It is necessary for the development of the gastrula that a force should act in the direction of the arrow in Fig. 2. Growth, cellular multiplication and reproduction are manifestations of etheric forces, but in gastrula formation we see a new phenomenon, a new force, different from the etheric forces, which does not exist in the plant. After having caused this invagination and formed for itself a cavity, this force establishes itself within—in a nest, as it were. This constitutes a third element in the animal—the first two being the physical body and the etheric body—and this anthroposophy calls the soul body or astral body, the reason for which name we will return to later. All that is connected with feeling—instincts, desires passions, attractions and repulsions—is an expression of the astral body, the psyche, the content of the soul.

What the external world presents is interiorized by the astral body and is then exteriorized in the form of movement. There is in this, as it were, a kind of respiratory movement, an alternation between interiorization, a form of 'sympathy', and exteriorization, a form of 'antipathy', which leads one to the concept that air is involved in these processes. Just as the etheric body has need of the liquid element as a medium, so the astral body can act only through the gaseous element.

We have suggested the possibility of developing latent faculties which permit us to perceive the etheric body. If we continue to develop these faculties by means of appropriate training, we can likewise arrive at 'perception' of the astral body, not only by its manifestations apparent to the senses, but also in its intrinsic reality.[4]

We have seen that the etheric body works in opposition to the laws of the physical world, and that the astral body is similarly opposed in its turn to the etheric, but this latter opposition manifests itself on another level. In imposing a change in direction on the etheric body, the astral body restrains it, and this in turn brings new properties into the material substance of the body.

The well-known experiment on the chicken's heart by A. Carrel can help us to grasp this action of the astral body.[5] The isolated cell of the chicken's heart is no longer under the influence of the chicken's animating astral body. So what happens to it? It multiplies to form a mass which resembles the morula and the life which manifests in it is purely vege-tative, purely etheric (though really a truncated etheric), whereas its reactivity and cellular differentiation has dis-appeared.

The animal is, as we have already pointed out, a horizontal being, whilst man has become a vertical being. Compared with the vertical plant, the animal has achieved a rotation of 90° to become horizontal. Man has rotated 180° relative to the plant. The idea of man as a superior animal is one of the main errors of materialistic science impeding the development of our knowledge of man. Just as there is a decisive step between animal and plant, so there is between man and animal. The upright posture of man is only a particularly striking manifestation of this step forwards. There are animals, of course, capable of standing upright for a relatively short period, but the upright position demands from them an effort which they are incapable of sustaining for long. In man, on the other hand, his weight is so perfectly balanced that only the minimum of effort is necessary for him to stand upright. His tendency to stand vertically is evident in his standing posture in general, and manifest in the smallest detail of his skeleton. This can be clearly seen if we compare the skeleton of a man with that of an anthropoid ape. For example, in the ape the heaviness of the skull has to be compensated for by the powerful musculature of the neck. In man, on the other hand, the head is balanced on the spinal column, which is almost straight whilst preserving only a slight reminder of snakelike sinuosity, just sufficient to give it a necessary suppleness.

Speech is another purely human characteristic. Animals cry out, but only man speaks (note that the parrot merely imitates a noise which is meaningless to it). Reactions in animals are in some degree automatic and can even be wholly induced in them by training. Human language is not present at birth. It has to be learnt, just as we learn to stand upright, by repeated effort. The third faculty which belongs to man alone is thinking, which also has to be learnt, and we are always astonished when we discover that a child is beginning to think independently.

An animal is entirely dependent on external stimuli and its own instincts. The circumstances in which it finds itself at a given moment recall past circumstances. Only man can voluntarily recall the past and immerse himself in it of his own accord. Man can also commune with himself and observe his own thought. He can become the object of his introspection, and can also call himself by that little word which he would not be able to use for anyone else—I. He is not only conscious of the external world around him as is the case in the animal, but he also differentiates himself from this exterior world and is conscious of himself. This I, this ego, is not an abstraction as certain philosophers have conceived it to be, but an entity as real as are the physical body, the etheric body and the astral body; it is the *human spirit*. From it emanates that force which gives our organism its individual human form, the force which impels the child to stand upright, to speak and to think. Like the other bodies it works through a medium—warmth. If it were possible for us to isolate the heat of our organism, we should see that it is not the same throughout the body, but that it displays a structure, an organization (an organization, moreover, that can be made partially evident by infra-red photography). So it is perfectly justifiable to speak of a 'heat organism' through which the ego acts. Similarly the astral body has an 'air organism' for its medium and the etheric body a 'water organism'. We can sum all this up in the table below.

CONSTITUENT ELEMENTS OF THE HUMAN BEING	ORGANIC MEDIUM	NATURAL ELEMENTS
Ego or human spirit	Heat organism	Fire
Soul body or astral body	Air organism	Air
Etheric body	Water organism	Water
Physical body	Mineral organism	Earth

We thus have our physical body in common with the mineral kingdom, our etheric body in common with the vegetable kingdom and our astral body with the animal kingdom. Only we, however, possess an ego or human spirit.

Each kingdom is in a certain sense opposed to the preceding one, and this opposition is present between the animal kingdom and man. An animal is entirely subject to its instincts and impulses. Man, thanks to his ego, has the capacity to resist them. He has in himself the *potential* for freedom. He can make a choice in accordance with a moral ideal. This liberty is not a natural endowment (for in that case it would no longer be a liberty!), but it is possible for him to win it by his own will. We have passions, impulses and instincts in common with all human beings. It is in the way that we govern them that we distinguish ourselves from each other.

Animals within the same species are far less individualized and unique than human beings, each of whom is a separate entity quite unlike any other. This is shown in our physical constitution, in our blood, for example, which is never identical with that of any other person. This individuality is present down to fine details such as the fingerprints. Nevertheless it is not the physical body as such that assures the permanence of these individual characteristics, for it merely receives the imprint of the ego through the intermediary of the astral and etheric bodies. In fact, the substance of the physical body is entirely renewed every seven years, and would thus be incapable of maintaining the human structure in its integrity without the action of the ego on the physical body through the mediation of the astral and etheric bodies. This renewal of the substance of the body over seven years was repeatedly stressed by Rudolf Steiner, but it has only very recently been possible to prove this, using radioactive elements. In spite of this renewal, we maintain the certain knowledge of our identity. Our substance changes, our appearance gradually alters and our mental content is modified, but nevertheless we do not doubt for a minute that we have remained the same individual, rich in all the memories gathered through the course of our existence.

These four constituent elements maintain more or less close connections with each other. The physical body and the etheric body, closely bound together, are almost exactly coincident in space and are only separated at death. They form the lower *physico-etheric complex*. The *higher complex*— the astral body and the ego—similarly maintain a close union, but it would be inexact to apply a spatial idea to this union, such as we conceive it in the material world; and instead of this we must substitute the degree of consciousness. The connection between the higher complex on the one hand and the lower on the other is less close and subject to variation. The higher complex detaches itself from the lower during sleep, and what remains in the bed can be compared with a plant, with the difference, however, that in man the higher elements have left a residual impulse in the etheric body. This impulse gradually becomes weaker and, since the human being cannot live without it, it becomes necessary for the ego and the astral body to incarnate anew in the lower complex; in other words, we wake up again. Waking consciousness and consciousness of the self are closely bound up with the presence of the ego and the astral body in the lower physical and etheric complex. When at death the etheric body also leaves the physical body, the latter returns to the mineral world, submitting exclusively to its influences, and disintegrates.

2.

THE HUMAN TRIAD

In getting to know the supersensible elements of man, we have taken a first step. We must now study the relationship between these elements and the different regions of the physical body.

Observation leads us to discern a polarity between the higher and lower parts of the organism. The almost perfectly spherical shape of the skull at the upper pole contrasts with the radiating structure of the limbs. The bones of the skull constitute a solid envelope surrounding the soft parts, while in the limbs it is, on the contrary, the hard parts which occupy the centre. In his head man is an invertebrate, but in his limbs a vertebrate. The radiating character of the limbs becomes even clearer when we count the bones: one for the thigh, two for the leg and five for the extremities. These two poles do not by themselves make a human being. They still need a middle part, a uniting element, without which the contrasting poles could not exist. This unifying element is the chest region or thorax. Considered as a whole, the thoracic cage possesses something of the spherical character of the head while each rib, taken separately, recalls the protraction of a limb. The thoracic cage also enfolds the soft parts, but is itself sur-rounded by important muscles. The spinal column, con-sidered as a whole, is an elongated structure surrounded by muscles like a limb, while each vertebra, taken separately, is a small skull enveloping the soft parts of the spinal cord.

We find again in physiology, in the functional, what we discover in anatomy. The bones of the skull, apart from the lower jaw, are immobile in relation to each other, while at the opposite pole the bones of the limbs are extremely mobile. The bones of the thoracic cage are only partly mobile and do not have the same freedom of movement as the limbs. Their movements are rhythmical just like those of the organs that they shelter; and so we call this middle region the rhythmical region.

The head's cephalic pole is a centre of absorption. Light, sounds, air and nourishment penetrate there. At the other extremity we encounter dispersion in the centrifugal motion of the excretions. Between the two we find harmonization, the re-establishment of equilibrium between the upper and the lower poles. The nerve-sense system is concentrated primarily at the cephalic pole and is the instrument of feeling, thought and consciousness. The lower pole is that of movement, of metabolism (which involves movement) and of exchanges. This is as true of the muscles as of the digestive apparatus. The entire metabolic system is the instrument of the will. In harmonizing the upper pole and the lower, in forming a bond between thinking and willing, the rhythmic system is the instrument of feeling or affect.

Man is thus a threefold being, but the above description is only a rough approach to the reality, for we can recognize this threefold division in all degrees, in all regions, in all organs and in each component part, however small it may be. Thus in the head the spherical element of the upper pole, with its contents of nervous substance, predominates only in the skull. The lower jaw, with its mobility, its muscles and its salivary digestive glands, recalls the lower pole. The nose also recalls the rhythmical system with which it communicates by means of the respiratory tract, just as the mouth communicates with the digestive apparatus. Nevertheless the dominant note of these three aspects of the head remains the spherical, cephalic, nerve-sense pole. We find these three stages again at the lower pole, though with an inverted dominance. Thus the femur has a head connected with an elongated part, the limb proper, by a neck which constitutes a middle zone. In the foot the rotundity of the heel recalls the cephalic pole, and the toes recall the radiating character of the limbs.

But man is an extremely complex being, and the study of the foot from the point of view of its threefoldness gives us an example. If the heel by its rounded shape recalls the cephalic pole, by its function, that is to say when it makes vigorous contact with the earth, it makes us think of the voluntary element of the lower pole. This is also accentuated when anger makes us stamp our feet. The toes, on the other hand, if they are 'limbs' in their structure, in the richness of their nerve fibres and in their function of feeling the way, belong to the nerve-sense system. Here we have a sort of paradox, a dissociation between form and function.

Such apparent contradictions are frequently found when studying the human being. It is very important to fathom their meaning. The paradox can be resolved in the case of the foot if one pictures to oneself what a sensory process is as a whole. Perception is a purely nerve-sense act, but in the toes that feel the way there is a 'will to perceive', a process which is both voluntary and sensory. In a way it is through the wish to perceive, to touch and to feel the ground, that the nerve-sense apparatus has been impelled to extend its ramifications right to the extremities of the limbs. This participation of the will is found also in other sensory activities when we *direct* a glance or *lend* an ear.

We can make similar observations in regard to the hand. Sometimes it closes to form a fist—a head in miniature—symbol of the will, often a will opposed or restrained, which explains the 'cephalic' appearance of the fist. And at other times it opens out into a sensory organ which touches. Or again it becomes a rhythmical instrument of social contact when one shakes hands with a neighbour.

All the above shows us how necessary it is for us to maintain a dynamic way of thinking if we wish to understand the human being. Thinking that is too systematized and drily intellectual is incapable of this. It merely dissects and apprehends what is dead, just as the chemist analysing a living substance begins by killing it!

In studying successively the nerve-sense pole, the metabolic or motor-digestive pole and the intermediary rhythmic system we have also divided up the human being, but in fact he is a whole and we must now reconsider him as such.

When we place a little sugar on our tongue we experience a sensation—that of sweetness. A nerve-sense process is involved which makes us become aware of a quality belonging to the substance placed on the tongue. But this is only part of the process. In reality the whole organism participates in this process and gets ready to receive the sugar, to transform it, to digest it and to transport it to where the organism has need of it. But only what takes place in the nerve-sense sphere reaches our consciousness. Once past the pharynx, everything that takes place is below the level of consciousness. Conversely, everything that takes place in the motor-digestive pole is reflected in the cephalic pole. We are thus conscious of the result of our movements and this permits us to control them.

A condition of normality implies an equilibrium between these two poles. If one of them has the tendency to make its activity prevail over the other, it is necessary for equilibrium to be re-established, a task which falls on the rhythmic system whose principal organ is the heart. This last acts both as a nerve-sense organ, perceiving what comes from above or below, and also as a barrage which dams up and canalizes the flow of blood in order to harmonize the two opposing tendencies. The mechanical notion which likens the heart to a pump is one of the great hindrances to progress in the knowledge of the physiology of the circulation of the blood. This prejudice is so strongly held that it is extremely difficult for people to rid themselves of it.

In his 'course for doctors' (1920)[1] Rudolf Steiner says:

There is an interaction in the first place between the liquefied foodstuffs and the air absorbed into the organism by breathing. This process is intricate and worth attention. There is an interplay of forces, and each force before reaching the point of interplay accumulates in the heart. The heart originates as a 'damming up' organ between the lower activities of the organism, the intake and assimilation of food, and the upper activities, the lowest of which is respiratory. A damming up organ is inserted and its action is therefore a product of the interplay between the liquefied foodstuffs and the air absorbed from outside. All that can be observed in the heart must be looked upon as an effect, not a cause, as a mechanical effect to begin with.

It is only very recently that this concept of the heart as an organ of equilibration has been able to be verified, and this has happened in two different ways. Professor Manteuffel has carried out experiments on dogs in which he bypassed the circulation from the heart.[2] He showed that the flow per minute was thereby considerably increased. If the heart were a pump one would have observed a diminution or even a stoppage of the circulation. Children affected by certain cardiac malformations also show a considerably increased circulatory flow. Professor Manteuffel cites the case of a little girl of nine years of age, weighing twenty-five kilos, whose circulatory flow per minute measured 11.3 litres. Sixteen days after the operation, carried out in the USA, it was 1.45 litres, which is normal. Other evidence points in the same direction. Moreover, embryologists know very well that the circulation of the blood precedes the existence of a heart and heart beats. We shall see subsequently how greatly the fact of envisaging the heart as an organ of equilibration can be fruitful from the point of view of the treatment of cardiac complaints. In any case, if one wishes to make a comparison of the heart with a machine it should be with a hydraulic ram, rather than with a pump.

Let us now attempt to examine the activities of the organism's two poles. We have defined the lower as being that of movement and metabolism (which is itself a movement since it involves an exchange of substances). In it we find an intense vitality, and consequently a corresponding activity of the etheric body. The constant regeneration of the cells of the intestine and cellular multiplication in the reproductive organs are pre-eminently etheric processes and manifestations of life. At the nerve-sense pole, on the contrary, it is the processes of death which dominate. This state of affairs attains its culmination in the nerve cell which is incapable of regeneration. One has the impression that it would need little to make it die altogether. Is that to say that the etheric forces are absent from the upper pole?

It is here that the law of compensation, of which we have spoken before, intervenes. Those etheric forces which have separated from the nerve-sense organs have become available on another plane, that of thinking. All those faculties of regeneration and of form production, the mobility, the infinite variety of forms which characterize life, and the etheric forces, which are at its source, we find active in our thinking. In thinking we can create the most diverse images, shape them, link them together, cut them off and make them grow again with that multiplicity of appearances which we find in the vegetable world. That is what has become of our etheric forces at the upper pole. At the lower pole they induce an intense vitality of the metabolism, while at the upper pole they no longer act in modelling substances but in building up thoughts and linking them together. The natural consequence of this is a much less intimate bond between the etheric body and the physical body at the upper pole. These etheric forces have been metamorphosed and put at the disposal of the astral or soul body and the ego, and intervene on the psycho-spiritual plane (see table on p. 89).

The foodstuffs which we absorb are substances which are foreign to our organism, and it is necessary for them to be divested of their own etheric force for the organism to be able to absorb them. This takes place in the digestive tract. There the foodstuffs are broken down and deprived of their foreign etheric forces under the influence of astral forces emanating from the upper pole. In striving to overcome these foreign etheric forces, the organism strengthens itself also, and this is the essential point of the alimentary process. It is not so much the substances which are significant as the forces over which they are victorious.

After being broken down, these substances pass through the wall of the digestive tract and undergo a new process of elaboration. They are then imbued with truly human etheric and astral forces. We thus see that the astral body acts in a contrary manner at the two poles of the organism. It induces the disintegrative processes from the cephalic pole and the building up processes from the metabolic pole, while at the level of the rhythmic system, astral forces constantly fluctuate between the two tendencies.

We have seen how the astral body has need of a medium, the gaseous element, in order to act. Under normal conditions this gaseous element is not free at the lower pole but in a state of solution in liquids. At this level the astral body is also closely bound to the organism. The astral body is able to partially free itself because it has its gaseous medium free within the lung. It is because the astral body is no longer so involved with metabolic processes that it becomes at this level available for the emotional life. We understand now why the latter is so closely bound up with our rhythmic system; for our emotional life is itself a perpetual swinging between the two poles of sympathy and antipathy, a respiratory process of the soul.

If the astral body, and also the ego, induce at the metabolic pole processes in which they are intimately involved, it is quite a different matter at the nerve-sense pole. Here, after elaborating the sense organs 'in their own image', they have withdrawn from them and made themselves into a kind of mirror. It is this which makes perception and the taking hold of conscious perceptions possible. If the astral body and the ego remained active in these organs, perception and waking consciousness would be impossible. It is absolutely necessary that our nerve-sense organs should remain free to receive external impressions. We have seen that the astral forces descending from the upper pole induce processes of disintegration in substances absorbed. At the upper pole these same forces cause breakdown of the substance of the organs themselves each time they come into play, indeed at the actual time of the phenomenon of perception and the exercise of consciousness. Through the action of the ego it is even more than a disintegration; it is a true death process which is provoked. The reason that the organs are not destroyed is because the part of the etheric body which has remained bound to them at once regenerates what has been damaged. We find here again a conflict between the lower physico-etheric complex and the higher astral and ego complex.

The processes of consciousness are intimately associated with a diminution of vitality; and we can now understand more easily why life has so largely withdrawn itself from our sense organs, why the nerve does not regenerate and why the eye resembles a piece of physics apparatus. It can happen, nevertheless, that metabolic processes can manifest themselves where they are absent under normal conditions. That is what happens in, for example, inflammation of the eye or ear; in such a condition these organs become incapable of their function of perception. Even a simple conjunctivitis considerably disturbs vision, and an ear affected by otitis media no longer hears effectively. This opens up new horizons for us in our ideas of illness.

3
HEALTH AND DISEASE

It is not really possible to arrive at an understanding of illness by dissecting a corpse, for the post-mortem examination can disclose only the final results of disease, not the causes. A fuller understanding of illness can only be reached by observing it in the living.

It is characteristic of illness that it is accompanied by changes in our state of consciousness. Even a simple headache or an attack of gout entails a disturbance of consciousness, so that we feel unwell. It is in the nature of being ill that we become conscious of organic processes which normally pass unnoticed. The state of well-being is characterized by a total unawareness of what is happening in our organs, so that we become aware of their existence only when their function is disturbed. The processes of consciousness normally belong to our nerve-sense apparatus, i.e. to the cephalic pole, and that is their proper place. When consciousness develops at the metabolic pole or in the rhythmic system, it is the expression of a morbid or an anomalous state.

We have seen that the processes of consciousness involve the presence of an astral body and an ego, and are intrinsically connected with processes of physical breakdown and death. When nerve-sense processes become too dominant they begin to encroach on the rest of the organism, where they manifest as an abnormal state of consciousness. This can affect various areas in the form of simple discomfort, pain or cramps. In a similar way the metabolic or motor functions are hindered. The organism has the tendency either as a whole or in an isolated organ to become too much 'head', and the processes of consciousness and disintegration are intensified at the expense of those of growth and regeneration. We have received the fruit of the tree of consciousness and lost that of the tree of life. Illness thus appears as a displacement of the etheric or astral forces or a preponderance of one over the other. What was proper in one region of the organism manifests inappropriately elsewhere and becomes illness.

As long as the abnormal action of the astral and the ego affect the etheric body alone, we remain in the functional sphere, but if the abnormal action is sufficiently prolonged it can affect the physical body, stamping it like a seal on wax, and causing physical effects. These are the pathological effects revealed by post-mortem examination, which can clearly give rise to symptoms.

It may be possible that the etheric is sufficiently strong to compensate the action of the astral and the ego. In such a case the illness does not manifest even at a functional level but remains latent. It is only when a certain threshold is reached that the etheric body is no longer capable of re-establishing harmony and the illness becomes manifest.

In this view health is a precarious equilibrium which must constantly be re-established. The great fomenter of troubles is the astral body and the great healer our etheric body. This will not surprise us when we recall that the astral body is the bearer of our instincts, passions and impulses. We can also understand that man, in whom a part of the etheric forces has been diverted from the metabolic system to be placed at the service of thinking, is much more vulnerable than less evolved creatures in which etheric forces remain available for regeneration.

In dealing with the predominance of the astral we have only grappled with one aspect of illness, for the opposite can also occur. It can happen that the etheric forces which have become free can remain unutilized because the ego is not strong enough to metamorphose them into thought forces. These unused etheric forces then have the tendency to act on their own account, causing proliferation, abnormal vegetative processes or tumour formation.

We now face two divergent aspects of illness: in the first the etheric body is called upon excessively and the forces which are needed for regenerating the organism are in some degree withdrawn from it; and in the second the etheric forces which have become free remain unutilized and unfold their potential where they should not do so. This predominance of the etheric is, moreover, accompanied by a diminution of consciousness, by a certain degree of clouding of the mind.

An example of premature abstraction of etheric forces, which unfortunately is very common today, results from too early formal academic learning, which entails intellectual development before the necessary etheric forces have become free. It is perfectly possible to call on these forces prematurely in order to hasten intellectual development. But it is precisely in this that the danger lies, for it is easy to ignore the fact that this abstraction of etheric forces is made at the expense of health, even if the consequences do not appear immediately. The consequences may occur only much later, but they may often manifest throughout life.

This in principle seems all very simple. In practice, however, it is often very difficult to understand to which of the tendencies described above an illness should be ascribed, for the symptoms we observe are, in reality, the responses or reactions of the organism, and these may manifest in very similar ways, yet have quite contrary causes. Thus when the forces of the astral body originating in the cephalic pole are insufficient for breaking down the foodstuffs and for the removal from them of their innate etheric forces, incompletely changed foodstuffs remain from this process and then become a medium for pathological intestinal flora and fermentation and abdominal distension occurs. But it can also happen that the astral forces descend too forcefully, and processes which normally take place at the level of the lungs—the release of carbon dioxide—occur at the level of the stomach or even in the intestine. Then gas will collect in the stomach or intestine, giving rise to abdominal distension. This has to be distinguished from distension that is caused by fermentation.

It also happens that phases belonging to one tendency succeed those of the other, the second sometimes being a reaction to the first. We can observe this phenomenon by studying what happens in the case of a cut. In the first phase there appear pain and inflammation, expressions of an increased activity of the astral body (pain) and of the ego (heat). Then comes a phase of proliferation in which the etheric body regenerates the tissues destroyed, and finally a third phase of hardening and consolidation of the newly formed tissues in which the etheric partly withdraws again from the zone of cicatrization and the astral again intensifies its action, this being expressed for our consciousness by itching. If one or other of these phases is hindered, proper healing fails to occur. Thus, if the first phase is prolonged and the second cannot succeed it at the proper time, we notice that the wound is atonic and shows no tendency to heal. If, on the other hand, the second phase exceeds its bounds—and this is often a reaction to unwise use of disinfectants—we see the proliferation of fleshy granulations which often give rise to cheloids.

An illustration of a very important principle in practice is the occurrence, in many or most cases, of a polarity between the site where the symptoms appear and the region in which we must seek their cause. We can, for example, reflect on the hepatic aetiology of the dermatoses. We can also observe a polarity in a condition such as otitis media. This, with its inflammation, lysis of tissues and pus formation, is a metabolic process manifesting itself at the nerve-sense pole. Moreover, it is patients in whom the metabolic pole is predominant who are the most susceptible to this condition.

It is therefore essential to be able to assess symptoms at their true value and always to look for the disturbance which corresponds to them at the opposite pole.

The knowledge that a patient is suffering from pneumonia is not in itself an absolute indication for treatment. Present-day medicine in these cases prescribes antibiotics, which are in reality only palliative since they are aimed at the symptoms of the illness—the microbe infection. Suppression of the symptoms does not constitute a true cure and nearly always causes the illness to be turned inwards, so that it will have the tendency to manifest itself again in the same form or in another form, which is often more subtle and more chronic. Many doctors are aware of this and have noted lingering states of ill health following such conditions which have been 'repressed'.

But let us return to the subject of pneumonia and take as an example one stage in its development, that of pulmonary hepatization. This descriptive term expresses perfectly what actually happens—part of the lung takes on a consistency which would be normal if it were liver. It becomes an organ that in a way resembles the liver, which is an organ of metabolism. Processes that are normal in the liver have been displaced to a higher level, to that of the lung. No doubt the resemblance is not perfect, for the structure of the lung does not allow that. What takes place in the lung is only a copy of the liver process. If we are able in our treatment to dispel these metabolic processes that have been displaced into the lung and restore them to their normal place, we are likely to bring about a much more fundamental cure than we should by merely destroying the bacteria that have settled only secondarily in an organ which was already ill. This is actually possible. We can find these forces of reconstruction in antimony and in particular in *Tartarus stibiatus*, which has a regulating effect on liver function. We have here only partially considered one aspect of the illness as an example. A more detailed study would lead us to other remedies such as, for example, *Phosphorus* or *Ferrum phosphoricum*, but that would take us too far ahead for the moment.

This example should spur us on to try and understand for ourselves what happens in other situations from this wider viewpoint. Such connections between pathology and therapeutics cannot be discovered by intellectual thought alone. They call for meditative effort on the part of the doctor, for the development of a consciousness 'more widely awakened' than it is during our everyday life. This is not an easy path to take, but he who succeeds in following it, and achieves a conscious therapeutic intuition, will find revealed to him possibilities of healing which work more deeply than those which have so far been available.

Among the symptoms which we observe, those relating to the psyche are no less important than those which are revealed to us in relation to the physical body. The classification of illnesses into mental and physical is somewhat schematic and really only relates to the predominant symptom among those observed. The boundary between the two categories remains blurred. We have already seen that every disease is accompanied by modifications of consciousness and that no so-called mental illness exists which is not accompanied by physical changes. The body, or more exactly the physico-etheric complex, is the instrument of the astral-ego complex. How can the latter express itself through a defective instrument? It is in no way surprising, therefore, that psychological symptoms can help us to understand better what is taking place in the organism. Moreover, we shall see that there are psychological symptoms that are characteristically associated with malfunction of certain organs. We can, for example, distinguish different kinds of fears associated with different organs. Homoeopathic practitioners know this very well, having discovered it empirically. But empiricism, however fruitful it may be in practice, is unable to satisfy us on the plane of thought for which we are striving. We feel in the depths of ourselves a need to understand and to connect together our diverse observations. We are unable, nowadays, to be content with mere belief, tradition, dogma or theory, if it is not possible for us to illuminate it by our thought.

Having related illnesses to our states of consciousness, it would be justifiable to ask why the astral body bears in it such a morbid potentiality. The answer would be beyond the scope of a medical work, but those who are interested can find it in other anthroposophical works.[1]

4
HYSTERIA AND NEURASTHENIA

We have already shown that the relationship between the physical, the astral and the ego is not the same at the two poles of the organism.

At the lower pole, that of exchanges and of movement, the ego acts in close unity with the other bodies. It would be more exact to say that the ego's action on the organism is made *through*, or *through the mediation of*, the astral body, the etheric body and the physical body. This mediating action shows itself in the organism in processes of tissue formation, regeneration and vitalization carried by the bloodstream throughout the whole organism as far as the nerve-sense pole. The bloodstream is regulated and given rhythm by the heart and, although it is diffused throughout the body, it really has its origin in the metabolic pole.

At the nerve-sense pole, on the other hand, the different supersensible aspects are in some degree separated.[1] At this level the ego, instead of acting successively through the medium of the other bodies, unites directly with the organism. This direct action of the ego follows the nerve tracts, inducing processes of tissue breakdown and structural organization.[2]

The first current, arising from the metabolic pole, vivifies substances or 'etherizes' them while the second, arising from the nerve-sense pole, kills them and mineralizes them, and thus makes the processes of thinking and of conscious mental activity possible. What the second current arising from the upper pole has killed must be revitalized by the first current arising from the lower pole, otherwise the organism would perish. The two currents should work in a constant harmony brought about by the mediating action of the rhythmic system and in particular of the heart. To complete the picture we must point out that there are two more intermediary currents of attenuated breakdown and regeneration. So as not to get lost in detail, we can group these together with those described above.

The equilibrium between these different currents is not the same in all individuals, and the predominance of one or the other current will cause different morbid tendencies.

The breaking down processes induced by the upper currents play an important part in digestion. We have seen that foodstuffs have to lose their own characteristics in order to be allowed to pass through the wall of the digestive tract and must therefore undergo breakdown and almost disintegration. Let us assume that the upper currents are too weak to break down the foodstuffs completely. These will then tend to maintain their own characteristics within the organism, to behave there like foreign substances, so that the organism contains chemical and physical activities from the outer world. Rudolf Steiner has given the name of *hysteria* to disturbances resulting from the presence of these foreign forces in the organism. As used by him, this word does not denote only the mental and emotional symptoms, with which we are familiar, but also a whole group of disturbances, of which the hysteria described by psychiatrists is only the culminating point.

It can happen, on the other hand, that the upper currents, which bring about breakdown of form, are too intense. The ego uses up its effect at the nerve-sense pole to some degree and no longer has enough strength to bring about correctly, through the intermediary of the astral, etheric and physical bodies, the processes of regeneration and growth at the lower pole. The processes of death and breakdown take the upper hand and the organism then becomes too 'spiritual', one could also say too 'intellectual'. The resulting inadequate regeneration then shows itself as a tendency to accumulate waste products which are deposited in the organism and may themselves become foreign bodies. Rudolf Steiner chose the name of *neurasthenia* for this second variety of disturbance, in which the breaking down processes predominate. He used this term also in a wider sense than has been given to it by psychiatry.

It is very important to make a vivid picture for oneself of this polarity between the two morbid tendencies of hysteria and neurasthenia, for it is not too much to say that all illnesses have a leaning more or less towards one or other of these morbid tendencies.

It is not possible to observe these supersensible currents directly unless one has developed in oneself the faculties of clairvoyance, but one can observe their symptoms, that is to say the reactions of the organism to these processes. These are, however, infinitely varied and often misleading. The organism can react to a foreign body, for example, either by eliminating it by means of an inflammatory process or by encapsulating it through a process of sclerosis. Inflammation with its blood manifestations and its intense vital processes must be considered as a reaction which is 'hysterical' in nature, a fact which does not prevent it arising on occasion after a 'neurasthenic' condition. Sclerosis, on the other hand, with its processes of ageing, tissue breakdown, devitalization and accumulation of wastes, is a typically neurasthenic reaction. We can nevertheless find it in a subject of a hysterical type in whom the organism in some degree lacks reaction and is no longer capable of an inflammatory reaction. Knowledge of these phenomena allows one to develop an extremely flexible therapy, enabling one to support the organism's own efforts at healing and to avoid interfering with them.

In the light of the above, it is interesting to study a condition typical of one of these processes. When the breakdown of foodstuffs is insufficient, owing to weakness of the upper currents, substances may pass through the wall of the intestine still retaining their foreign character. A certain external, extra-human activity still holds sway in the interior of the digestive tract, even under normal conditions, but once substances pass through the wall of the intestine we are really inside man, where only 'human' processes should exist. Everything passing through the intestinal wall that is foreign then acts like a poison or toxin, which the organism then tries to eliminate. It does not always succeed in this, particularly if the liver is not functioning as it should. These toxins are then carried by the bloodstream to the nerve-sense pole which, in its turn, tries to 'digest' them, to complete what the digestive tract had been unable to do. The organs of the nerve-sense pole are not, of course, designed for this task, and the astral body and the ego, from this unaccustomed effort, become too closely associated with these organs. This unaccustomed contiguity shows itself in pain. We have now sketched a picture of migraine and we could elucidate all its symptoms as Husemann has done.[3]

We can now understand why it is that anything which diminishes the action of the astral body and the ego at the upper pole favours the development of migraine. Thus the menstrual period, which calls for an increased activity of the astral body and the ego at the lower pole, thereby detracting from the already inadequate forces of the upper pole, can be the precipitating cause of an attack. In cases of dietary excess the upper current is incapable of taking up its task properly, so that sufferers from migraine have an instinctive tendency to reduce their food intake. Strong emotions, arguments, mental overwork and the excessive quantity of sense impressions, which accompany modern life, call too much on the astral body and the ego and prevent them from carrying out their digestive task, and can in this way start off an attack of migraine. We note also that the action of the astral body and the ego are more intense at the upper pole in men and that men are, generally speaking, less liable to migraine than women in whom these elements are, on the contrary, more intimately united with the lower pole.

What therapy should one propose for this condition of a frankly hysterical type? At the time of attack the process is so far advanced that it is difficult to combat, but that does not mean that there is no possibility of alleviating it. I will mention one treatment which has sometimes enabled me to cut short a threatened attack—to inhale from a vessel containing mustard. Normally if one puts one's nose over a mustard pot one experiences a violent prickling sensation bringing on watering of the eyes. In an attack of migraine one can inhale from a mustard pot without it causing one any disturbance. The sulphurous emanations of the mustard redirect the astral body to its task, diverting the process towards a lower level; and as a result the pain abates somewhat.

One cannot talk of migraine without saying a word about aspirin and other analgesics. Certainly in a case of extreme need—such as sitting for an examination, for example—we are in practice obliged to have recourse to them. It is nevertheless important to know that analgesics hinder the action of the higher bodies on the nerve-sense organs, for this is the cause of their analgesic action. Their habitual use will, therefore, weaken the already failing upper currents in these patients, *increasing* the predisposition to attacks of migraine.

Rudolf Steiner, conscious of the social importance of this condition and the increasing frequency of its occurrence owing to the conditions of modern life, proposed a remarkable remedy for its treatment. This is Bidor (*Ferrum sulph.* 5%/*Silica* 5%/*Mel* 5% aa trit.). The combination of iron and sulphur acts on the meeting point between the digestive and respiratory processes. Sulphur, as we have already found with mustard, intensifies the metabolic processes. Iron stimulates the respiratory processes, which is one of the reasons for its presence in haemoglobin. By giving a combination of iron and sulphur we harmonize the metabolic and respiratory functions, and thus prevent the digestive functions from overflowing towards the upper pole. Silica, or quartz, is characterized by its form-giving forces. These forces, as we have seen, normally exist at the upper pole where they have been interiorized. By giving quartz we strengthen the upper, form-giving currents. A common simile can help us to grasp the action of this mineral and to recall the connection that exists between the form-giving processes and thinking—do we not talk of an idea being as clear as crystal? Mel, honey, calls especially on the forces of the ego. There is a strong connection between the human ego and the beehive which has the astonishing property of maintaining a constant temperature, a fact unique in the insect world.

Bidor 1% or 5% should be administered for periods of seven weeks, one tablet three times a day. Each course is followed by an interval of five weeks during which *Aurum* 10x can be given and also a course of treatment to improve liver functions. For this we prescribe Hepatodoron and *Chelidonium* comp. The seven-week courses of Bidor should be continued for months, even for two or three years, but a distinct improvement is usually noted after the first two weeks. One must have the patience to continue the treatment for a sufficient time if one wants to obtain a permanent cure. Obtaining a cure may also necessitate the patient changing his way of life and eating habits.

Migraine is one mode of reaction against foreign processes which penetrate into the organism. Matters do not always go as far as this and reactions can take place at a number of levels. Thus protein, which retains extra-human properties, may be eliminated by the kidneys, but this does not necessarily mean that the kidneys become diseased, though they could do so if this extra work is demanded of them for too long. The organism can also get rid of intolerable foreign materials by means of an acute inflammation, a sore throat for example, or by way of the skin in the form of eczema.

The direct action of the ego and the astral body on the organism necessarily entails a predominance of catabolic processes, giving rise to the appearance of inorganic or even mineral substances. The ego needs these mineral elements in small quantities for the processes of consciousness, but the remainder has to be revitalized by the etheric forces from the currents arising from the lower pole. In conditions of a neurasthenic type the excess of the processes of disintegration, as opposed to those of revitalization, leaves a residue which tends to be deposited as a foreign body which the organism then attempts to eliminate. It is these attempts at elimination, these reactions of the organism to the deposits, which produce the symptoms which we observe. A youthful organism has a greater tendency to react by an inflammation, so as to get rid of the foreign substance by means of pus formation. A sore throat or sinusitis is then a reaction to a process of the neurasthenic type. But in the long run, if the causes persist, the organism tires and resigns itself to the foreign presence, and is no longer capable of reacting by an inflammation. The foreign elements then tend to precipitate in the form of calculi, atheromatous plaques and tophi. In a general way, the organism becomes sclerotic. We are then confronted with morbid processes proper to an ageing organism.

There is still one method of defence remaining before the total resignation of the organism—encystment. In this process the organism makes a membrane which isolates the foreign body from the tissues. It is precisely because the human etheric forces can no longer penetrate it that something becomes a foreign body. These forces then concentrate themselves all the more strongly at its periphery and this shows itself by the formation of an *encysting membrane*.[4] Although less active than the process of inflammation, encystment nevertheless remains a method of defence for the organism. This explains why a tumour, which is itself usually the seat of foreign forces, is generally benign when it is well limited by an encysting membrane.

So far we have considered hysteria and neurasthenia under their organic or, we could say, their somatic aspects. Let us now try to realize why physical or functional symptoms sometimes seem to dominate, and at other times mental manifestations are most apparent.

To understand this it is necessary for us to come back to the idea of equilibrium, harmony and compensation, brought about by the rhythmic system between the upper and lower poles.

We do not observe any symptoms as long as this compensation is able to continue. If, however, it happens that one of the disturbing elements shows an abnormal intensity, then we may see functional conditions appear, in other words a dysfunction of the etheric body. If the causes persist and if the equilibrium cannot be re-established, the irregularities of the etheric body impress themselves on the physical body as a seal does on wax. Then we see the physical symptoms appear which can be revealed to us by palpation, auscultation, radiography, endoscopy and autopsy. We then have a temporary or permanent lesion of the organ.

But it can also happen that the condition, although persistent, is not severe enough to give rise to functional signs; that is, it does not manifest itself on the etheric plane. The condition nevertheless exists in the etheric body even if it does not become manifest there. As Rudolf Steiner has said, the etheric then imprints its seal on the physical organ in a more superficial and less evident way, but this prevents the organ from correctly fulfilling its function as a 'mirror', or instrument, of the soul. It is as if this mirror had lost its clarity and no longer allows the astral body and the ego to 'reflect' themselves there correctly; and this gives rise to distorted and abnormal mental symptoms. Such manifestations are characteristic of the particular organ damaged, and of its functions. They can appear separately, but it is not uncommon to see them alternate with corresponding organic diseases.

It is important to note this contrast, that deep lesions of organs, those that we recognize on physical examination, hardly ever produce mental disturbances. They are in a way sited 'behind the mirror' and do not alter its reflecting power for the soul. One could also say that the deep lesion constitutes a kind of diversion onto the physical plane, so that we often see mental illness diminish or disappear when an organic condition develops.

Is it possible to demonstrate the superficial lesions of which we have just been speaking? In certain cases, yes, but it seems that our methods of investigation are not yet sufficiently refined to permit this in all cases.

Are we then still in a position to assert that these connections exist between organs and mental conditions? Without any doubt, for successful therapy furnishes indisputable confirmation of what spiritual research has taught us on this subject.

It is tempting to try to establish a kind of classification of conditions as hysterical or neurasthenic. I have been content to give the example of migraine, not in order to classify but to point out a line of thought. It is most important to try to discover in every case what is actually taking place. A ready-made classification would introduce the great danger of putting quite different conditions under one and the same heading, for it is not the name which we give to a condition that counts but the true understanding of the process involved in producing it. Certainly there are illnesses that are typical and we need schemas to help us retain certain details in our memory. We must train ourselves to consider the schemas only as props which we need for a certain time and subsequently relinquish. It is precisely by finding out what characterizes a patient of a general type that we arrive at an understanding of him as an individual.

These ideas will now guide us in the direction of therapy. It is possible here to give only a brief and general sense of this. When we have to deal with a patient of a hysterical type, we seek to strengthen the ego and the astral body in their upper currents, and this we can do with *Stibium*. Antimony, which crystallizes in fine radiating needles, has a form-endowing capacity particularly with regard to proteins. It can also act in the organism like the ego, so that it can for a while act as a substitute for the ego, thus allowing the ego itself time to recover its strength. We give it in the form of injections[5] of *Stibium praep.* 6x–10x.[6] Its combination with silver in the mineral dyscrasite is particularly useful in patients whose conditions are on the borderline between the mental and the physical. In these cases one should use it in high potency—in 30x. In acute manifestations of hysteria we make use of *Bryophyllum*, in injections of 3x to 5x, or in a 5% dilution. This plant of the *Crassulaceae* (Stonecrop) family has the property of being able to develop new plants from pieces of its leaves. This is evidence of great vitality and of extraordinary etheric forces. Introduced into the organism, these intense foreign etheric forces compel the etheric forces of man to a no less intense effort to take possession of them and hold them back in the lower part of the organism, and thus to prevent them from overflowing into the nerve-sense pole (for this reason the injections should be given in the thigh). For a treatment in greater depth one would prefer to use *Argentum per Bryophyllum*, a remedy obtained by 'dynamization' of silver through the plant.[7] We prescribe it in 0.1% or 1% by subcutaneous injection.

When the inadequate breakdown of proteins in the intestinal tract shows itself by the appearance of foreign proteins in the organism and their elimination by the kidneys, we prescribe *Pancreas* 3x/*Ferrum sidereum* 10x aa trit. Iron, the metal of incarnation, compels the ego to take possession of the organism more strongly.[8] In associating *Pancreas* with it, we direct its action towards an organ one of whose roles is particularly that of the breakdown of proteins. It is moreover recommended that this combination should be prescribed for convalescence from febrile diseases such as influenza, measles, scarlet fever, sore throats, etc.

In conditions of a neurasthenic type the basic remedy is *Phosphorus* in low dilution—5x or 6x. This element, which has the property of igniting spontaneously, acts as a guiding light to the ego and directs it in the darkness of the metabolic processes (and also the voluntary processes connected with metabolism). In cases of mental overwork we can advantageously substitute for it *Kalium phosphoricum* 6x. We must always bear in mind *Prunus spinosa*. This thorny plant with its short-lived bright blossom and its astringent fruit is rather the opposite of *Bryophyllum*, of which we have spoken above. If planted under an old apple tree it has the property of revitalizing it so that it becomes covered with leaves and fruit again. It possesses a revitalizing action also on the human organism. We can prescribe *Prunus spinosa* in the form of lukewarm baths (one teaspoonful of the extract is enough for a bath) or by subcutaneous injection in 3x strength.

When the astral body acts too intensively on the musculature, cramps develop. These can be effectively dealt with by an ointment containing copper (*Ungt. Cupri* 0.4%, to be rubbed into each leg on retiring at night). The same ointment can be applied to the abdominal wall in spasmodic constipation or the periumbilical colic of infants (the massage of the ointment should be carried out in a clockwise direction, always using very little of the ointment). The indications for the use of *Cupri* ointment are so numerous and varied that we can only give a general idea of its action here.

In conditions of a neurasthenic type one must also think of *Argentum*. One might be surprised to see it cited here, since we have already spoken of it in connection with hysteria. *Argentum* and *Phosphorus* are two remedies of opposite polarity and they should never be prescribed together. But they can perfectly well be used alternately, namely, *Argentum* with the waxing moon at night, and *Phosphorus* with the waning moon in the morning. This method of treatment gives particularly spectacular results when one is dealing with patients who are sensitive to the moon, and belong to one or other type. The rhythmical administration of these two remedies is a remarkable help when one wishes to re-establish harmonious equilibrium between functions which have become poorly connected to the physical organism.

5
SLEEPING AND WAKING

Many of our contemporaries in the Western world suffer from disturbances of sleep and, we should add, of disturbances of their waking life, for if they sleep badly at night they are often not properly awake during the day. But the problem of insomnia can be resolved only if we arrive at an understanding of the essential differences between sleeping and waking. This will also be an excellent opportunity for enlarging our knowledge of the nature of man.

In the alternation between these two states we immediately perceive a rhythmic process, an oscillation between two polarities: in one we are in command of our full consciousness and in the other we have no consciousness. There exist between these two poles intermediate states such as daydreams and dreams proper which are really gradations tending to some degree towards one or other of these poles.

In the waking state we have perceptions and mental images, we experience feelings and we can manifest our will. We feel ourselves to be beings distinct from the exterior world and distinct from other beings as individuals. Moreover, when we wake up we have an impression of continuity or, more accurately, an absolute certainty of being the same person as the one who fell asleep the night before, with the same content of consciousness (increased incidentally by the content of our dreams).

All this implies that when we are awake our astral body and our ego interpenetrate with the lower bodies (etheric and physical). What we feel from the fact of having awoken cannot be expressed in a logical manner in rational terms. We can have consciousness of it only by observing ourselves from within, i.e. in 'contemplating' ourselves. This attitude allows us the possibility of a path of knowledge not proceeding via the senses, like the external sciences, but which is nonetheless viable. We can very well have the opposite experience—by observing another person who is asleep. We can see his exterior form, we can weigh it and measure it, and we are therefore in the presence of a physical body; but we can also observe many manifestations which make us distinguish between someone who is asleep and someone who is dead. We witness, as we do in the plant, a mass of vital phenomena, which oblige us to infer the presence of an etheric body in addition to the physical body.

But nothing reveals to us the presence of the ego or even that of the astral body in someone who is asleep. We are therefore obliged to admit that the ego and the astral body have left the lower bodies during sleep and have in some manner become detached. It is now possible for us to realize why the higher elements, deprived of the instrument which the physical and etheric bodies constitute for them, are unable to recall what they have been able to experience when outside them during sleep. Certain materialistic trends of thought would have us believe that, because operations on the brain are capable of modifying our states of consciousness, mental activity is merely a secretion of that organ. This would be as absurd as suggesting that time no longer existed because we had broken our watch.

This somewhat schematic comparison of a sleeping person with a plant must not be pushed too far. Man is an extremely complex being and the schemas which we present can only be stepping-stones towards a more detailed understanding.

We saw in the preceding chapter that the astral body does not act in the same way at both the upper and lower poles. It has a breaking-down action from the nerve-sense pole, which

forms a basis for the processes of consciousness, and a
building-up, synthesizing action from the digestive pole. Only
that part of the astral body connected with the nerve-sense
system is separated from the lower bodies during sleep. The
other part remains associated with the digestive pole and has
in fact a more intimate relationship with the lower elements.
The processes of breakdown necessary for consciousness
being in abeyance, the processes of regeneration are all the
more active. All these phenomena can be directly observed by
the clairvoyant. In the absence of this gift we can note only
the external manifestations of the sleeping and waking states.
What has been described above will nevertheless allow us to
understand them better.

One generally thinks that the desire to sleep is due to
tiredness, but this is inaccurate. One can be very tired without
having the desire to sleep and, on the other hand, have the
desire to sleep without being really tired. Expressed in this
way, this may seem to be a play on words, for tiredness and
the desire to sleep are closely related concepts without precise
limits. However, what we experience as the desire to sleep is
really only the need of the higher bodies—the astral and the
ego—to separate themselves from the lower—the physical
and etheric. With the help of certain drugs like coffee we can
delay this need and make the sensation of tiredness disappear
for a certain time. With the help of other drugs we can exert
the opposite effect.

After the ego and a part of the astral body separate from
the lower bodies during sleep, they incarnate in them once
more on waking. If this incarnation is hindered for some
reason, we wake up badly and experience a feeling of tiredness (which can quite easily disappear after some time even
without resting). Generally speaking, we can say that
insomnia results from the upper elements having difficulty in
separating themselves from the lower. The causes of this

situation are many and various and we shall study some of them. This will guide us towards the possible ways of treating the condition.

When an organ is damaged for any reason, a disharmony arises between the physical body and the etheric body. This entails a more intense action of the astral body on the etheric body, so as to impel the latter to repair the damage. It can even happen that the astral body acts directly on the physical body and this will then show itself in pain and cramps. Pain is, in fact, a conscious expression of this over-activity of the astral body. It is obvious that a more intense union of the astral body with the lower elements at any point in the organism hinders its detachment from the physical and etheric which is necessary for sleep. The astral body and the ego remain caught up by the etheric and physical bodies at the site of the injury or disturbance. Such a union can, nevertheless, remain below the level of consciousness or fail to be perceived by consciousness owing to a nerve lesion (e.g. a devitalized tooth) and pain is then not experienced. We know also that certain organs, even when badly damaged, are not painful.

One must always question patients very precisely about their sleep. It can happen that, because attention is focused elsewhere, one omits to do this and then subsequently a patient whom one had treated successfully for a quite different condition informs us that his insomnia has disappeared. This is proof of the advantage of treating causes rather than just symptoms. It is very important to know the way in which a patient goes to sleep and how he wakes up, and about the quality of his sleep and of his waking state. Some patients are really properly awake only towards the evening, while others in contrast are full of animation from the moment they leap out of bed but are incapable of keeping awake in the evening. All these signs help one to grasp the relationships between the different sheaths of the ego which the astral, etheric and physical bodies form.

In training ourselves to decipher the disharmonies which can show themselves between the different bodies we shall become capable of establishing the truly causal therapy that should be the aim of all true medicine.

Conditions giving rise to insomnia often take a very long time to imprint themselves on the physical body and can remain for years in the functional sphere (that of the etheric). In such a patient, for example, disturbances of sleep may appear some time after a sore throat, accompanied perhaps by a fleeting albuminuria. This is on such a slight scale that laboratory analyses and functional tests may well reveal nothing. We should nevertheless think of the kidneys, prescribe *Equisetum* 6x and see everything restored to order again after a time. In another patient who wakes up regularly at three in the morning we shall suspect a hepatic lesion. We shall prescribe him Hepatodoron three times a day before meals to restore his liver functions, and perhaps also *Chelidonium* compound which acts particularly on the biliary function (ten drops after meals in half a glass of warm water or in an infusion). He should also be given hot compresses over the liver with an infusion of milfoil (or yarrow) after the midday meal; and we shall have the surprise of seeing the patient, who has probably been rather depressed, regain his spirits and his sleep.

It is as well to know that these insignificant lesions can sometimes continue to exist for years, and mar the life of these patients, whose complaints are often dismissed as imaginary when only a little attention and compassion are needed in order to help them. The kidneys and the liver are not of course the only organs to be suspected, and I have chosen them only as examples, for any organ can be involved. We shall consider later certain mental symptoms which may point us to certain organs. It should also be remembered that insomnia can be the first symptom of some more serious condition. We often meet with it in cancer patients in the period before the development of the tumour. In that case we obtain excellent results with injections of Iscador (fermented mistletoe, *Viscum album*), thus confirming the precancerous nature of the insomnia. We shall have occasion to return to this subject.

A discord between the physical and the etheric, which is not localized but is particularly stubborn, can arise as the result of a mental shock which should be sought for very carefully in a patient's medical history. In this case we prescribe *Argentum* 6x by mouth or better by subcutaneous injection, preferably given during the period of the waxing moon. If the shock took place a very long time ago, we shall use higher potencies (15x or 20x), but it is better in principle to start with 6x. *Argentum* is the remedy for the etheric body and it is often good to start with several injections of *Argentum* before proceeding to some other treatment. When a treatment that appears to us to have been carefully chosen shows itself to be ineffective, we can also prescribe a course of *Argentum* and then resume the previous treatment, which will become effective after *Argentum* has summoned the etheric forces.

Before finishing our consideration of physical lesions let us mention cold which can also be a cause of insomnia. Cold can result in true damage to our 'heat organism', preventing the astral body and the ego from detaching themselves. We know that cold feet hinder sleep. What is less well known is that a mattress which is insufficiently insulating leads to a progressive cooling down of the body, and can be a cause of early waking. Putting one or two *woollen* blankets over the mattress is enough to restore normal sleep. For patients suffering from cold feet one prescribes bathing the feet with hot and cold water alternately (1 minute in hot water and 15 seconds in cold water alternately, a dozen times), followed by gentle massage of the legs with copper ointment (*Ungt. Cupri* 0.4%). Excessive heat can naturally also disturb sleep, but patients are generally more conscious of this. Let us recall once more hunger and hypoglycaemia as a cause of early waking (which makes one think that the glass of sugared water our grand-mothers gave us did not rest on imagination alone).

In contrast, excess of food is itself a frequent cause of insomnia or, more exactly, of not sleeping well. When we eat a lot, we demand a particularly strong effort on the part of the digestion and call strongly on the forces breaking down the food which arise from the upper pole. It is not surprising that in such circumstances the detachment of these forces from the physical and etheric bodies is hindered. That over-eating is accompanied at the same time by a feeling of drowsiness is in no way paradoxical, since the forces used by the digestion are not fully available at the nerve-sense pole for the processes of consciousness. Under these circumstances we can neither be properly awake nor find peaceful sleep. There is a displace-ment of the astral which is in a sense the opposite of detachment. It can also happen that foodstuffs, as we have seen in migraine, pass through the intestinal wall without having lost all their 'external' forces. They then carry over with them their foreign characteristics into the interior of the organism, and what has not been completed in the digestive tract now has to be carried out by organs which are not properly equipped for such activity. The astral body and the ego are then drawn in an abnormal manner into these organs and this will hinder their detachment for sleep. As we found earlier, a similar process occurs in sufferers from migraine. It is understandable that there are also those who suffer from 'sub-acute migraine', in whom insomnia can be the main symptom. We treat these patients like those suffering from migraine with Bidor.

What has been stated above will give us a better understanding of the constitutional type of insomnia which can be met with in patients of the hysterical or neurasthenic types. In the latter, as we have seen in the preceding chapter, the union between the ego and the astral body in the nerve-sense system is too intense and it is, therefore, in no way surprising that these bodies have difficulty in detaching themselves. But these patients may show yet another characteristic symptom—they do not wake properly in the morning. If we observe them carefully, we find that this incomplete waking consists less in a lack of consciousness—their thinking is generally active enough although scattered—than in their inability to undertake anything. In order to understand these people properly we can make use of a simile, that of an archer whose right hand—the active side—holds the string of the bow which represents the will forces, while the left hand, which directs the arrow, can be likened to the thinking forces originating from the nerve-sense pole which direct the will towards a goal. These two forces are expressions of the ego at different levels of the organism. It is the right hand, the will forces, which does not wake up in the neurasthenic. His head is awake, but his ego does not succeed in taking possession of the metabolic pole, the seat of will. Such a patient will thus have many fleeting ideas, but his thinking, in order to be concentrated properly, needs the help of the will. In this situation he is incapable of undertaking anything constructively.

Phosphorus in low dilution (5x–6x) acts on the ego like a light to someone lost in the night, guiding it towards the lower pole and compelling it to incarnate better there. It acts on the patient's will like the Promethean fire brought to earth.

By helping the patient to take proper possession of his body in the morning, we make it easier for him as a counter-effect to get off to sleep at night. This shows us once again the importance of the rhythmic aspect of the organic functions.

We can ask ourselves with regard to phosphorus what would be the action of a very high dilution, such as 25x for example. This question equally concerns the treatment of insomnia, for if in 5x dilution this substance concentrates the ego in the lower pole, in high potencies it disperses it and draws it into cosmic spaces. We can therefore prescribe *Phosphorus* 25x at night to help a patient fall asleep.

As the opposite of the slender neurasthenic we have the hysteric of a rather pyknic constitution with a predominance of the digestive pole. If we resume our comparison with the archer it will be his right hand, his will forces, which will predominate. These will have a tendency to act without proper control, often to no purpose (cf. Chapter 4). Precisely because they are weak at the upper pole, the astral body and the ego will tend to stick fast, like an alpine climber who feels his strength weaken and fastens himself to one spot with crampons. The astral and ego forces rising from the lower pole, because they have fastened themselves on too closely to the physical and etheric, have difficulty in detaching themselves. This is the cause of insomnia in a person of hysterical type.

The remedy is, as we have seen (cf. Chapter 4) *Bryophyllum*, which is given as 5%, six drops at 6 p.m. In some patients the effects of this resistance to the exhaling of the ego and astral forces show themselves more in the rhythmic region in the form of difficulty in breathing, palpitations and a sensation of suffocation (precordial pain, on the contrary, is more a neurasthenic symptom). We prescribe for these patients Cardiodoron (*Primula* 2.5%/*Onopordon* 2.5%/*Hyoscyamus* 2.5% aa dil.) in order to harmonize the rhythmic functions (fifteen drops before the three main meals) or again *Aurum* 10x, ten drops at 9 p.m. Let us recall that the insomnia of hepatic origin, of which we spoke above, belongs especially to the hysterical type, although the indifferent nature of our present-day nutrition causes it also to be found in patients of the neurasthenic type. Conversely, insomnia resulting from an excessive nerve-sense excitation, which is characteristic of modern life, while affecting especially the neurasthenic type, also affects the hysterical type.

We have not yet suggested the use of any hypnotic drugs. It is usually possible to do without them, but one sometimes has to wean patients off them gradually, over a period of one or two weeks, if they have been taking them for a long time. If the habit is not of too long-standing, one can stop them abruptly, explaining to the patient that he must expect a few bad nights if he wishes to recover normal sleep. Detoxification of these patients should never be forgotten. It is always a good thing to remind them that the hypnotic which they have been taking no more procures for them a true sleep than a tablet of aspirin cures a carious tooth. The weaning from sedatives can usually be helped by a more symptomatic remedy such as *Avena sativa* comp. Patients who have more difficulty in relaxing and are anxious are given five drops of *Aconitum* 20x, and those who are very excited are given *Belladonna* 20x. On the other hand, *Coffea* 6x–12x works well in patients presenting mental hyperactivity with many fleeting thoughts.

In insomnia of young children, rickets should always be looked for; and the basic remedy for this condition is *Phosphorus* 5x, five drops in the morning. We meet again here the connection between *Phosphorus* and light. For children who have nightmares we give *Argentum* 6x trit., one tablet on going to bed during the waxing phase of the moon, alternately with *Phosphorus* 6x, five drops on waking during the waning phase of the moon. This remarkable treatment should be continued for several months and then consolidated by a course of *Ferrum praep.* 20x trit., a saltspoonful once or twice a day. I have often observed that children who have received large amounts of vitamin D as infants have been subject to nightmares. These children give the impression of being particularly hardened, appear older than their age, and have a premature intellectual development (which does not mean that they are more intelligent). In such cases *Argentum* can be replaced with advantage by *Argentum sulphuratum* 6x trit. Finally, a good remedy to help rather nervous children and infants to get off to sleep is *Chamomilla rad.* decoc. 6x dil., five drops twice daily before meals.

Plumbum melit. 12x or 20x trit. should always be thought of for elderly patients and this will be spoken of again under the subject of arteriosclerosis.

In a lecture course given for doctors and medical students in 1920[1] Rudolf Steiner foretold that we would see true epidemics of insomnia appear in the second half of the present century. Apart from the ill effects of modern life on man's natural rhythms there is a cause which one should not neglect. As Husemann[2] said: 'The person who sees his neighbour only as an aggregate of atoms cannot have the same conception of his real self. He thus arrives necessarily at a fundamental contradiction.'

Little by little the soul of such a person loses all possibility of experiencing the spiritual world, so that the spiritual realms become for such a soul like a desert. The fact of returning into the spiritual world on going to sleep—for the detachment of the astral body and the ego is, in reality, a return into the spiritual world—is felt by this soul as a descent into the void before which it draws back in terror. This unconscious fear prevents the detachment of the astral and ego so that the sufferer cannot sleep. It is not uncommon to find in such patients, who have often deeply plumbed the abyss of materialism, an unavowed and often unconscious nostalgia for spiritual nourishment. It is possible to help such patients by advising them to devote as little as five minutes each day to one of the meditations given by Rudolf Steiner. One must beware of any proselytism, if only out of respect for the freedom of the individual patient, and so one recommends these meditations as one would prescribe a remedy.[3]

Sleeping and waking now appear to us like a great respiratory rhythm—in the morning we breathe in our ego and astral body and in the evening we let them detach themselves again from the lower bodies which we leave in our beds. What happens on a large scale in the period of a day and a night is found again on a small scale in respiration. Each inhalation wakes us up a little, each exhalation sends us to sleep a little. All that is life is rhythm.

6

INFLAMMATION AND SCLEROSIS

Celsius distinguished inflammation by its four manifest-ations, which we all know: calor, dolor, tumor and rubor. We shall now enquire as to which of the elements that we have previously studied are related to these symptoms.

We have seen that the ego has the 'heat organism' for its physical medium. All heat processes in man are expressions of the activity of the ego so that we naturally relate the symptom *calor* to the ego. Pain is over-intense stimulation of con-sciousness, so that we can relate *dolor* to the astral body. *Tumor* is a swelling, a collection of liquid, and therefore expresses an action of the etheric body. We record *rubor*, redness, on the physical plane as the expression of the sub-stantial presence of blood. We can sum up the preceding in the following table:

Calor	expression of	ego
Dolor	" "	astral body
Tumor	" "	etheric body
Rubor	" "	physical body

Inflammation thus appears as the expression of the simultaneous activity of the four constituent elements, but of an ordered and organized activity in which the ego acts *through* the other three elements. In order to give a more exact concept of this phenomenon, we will modify the preceding table in the following manner:

Ego ——————————————————— → Calor
Ego → astral body ————————————— → Dolor
Ego → astral body → etheric body ————————— → Tumor
Ego → astral body → etheric body → physical body → Rubor

One could conceive an action by the etheric body in isolation, which would then express itself by a swelling, but this would be simply of a watery or lymphatic nature. The fact that the swelling is the result of an accumulation of blood is evidence of the action of the ego on the etheric body. This 'action in stages' reminds us of the process which we studied in relation to hysteria. Inflammation belongs really to the warm pole of the organism, to the metabolic pole, at whatever site it manifests. In so far as it is a pathological process, it is an intensification of the action of the ego working through the three bodies.

One might be surprised that there can likewise be inflammatory processes at the superior pole, but only if one does not take into account the fact that the superior pole is not exclusively nerve-sense activity but only predominantly so, just as the inferior pole, where metabolism predominates, also possesses nerves.

It remains for us to understand what the causes of inflammation are, and when it appears. The answer to this question is: every time a foreign body or foreign process manifests itself in the organism. The foreign presence may be of an accidental character (for example a splinter) but it is much more often the result of a dysfunction or of a disequilibrium, such as we studied in Chapter 4, para. 2. Foreign processes can also be a consequence of trauma, or of excessive cold or heat. A typical example of the inflammatory reaction following the introduction of a foreign mineral substance is the fever which is produced in an infant if one gives it a solution of 1% sea salt to drink. Inflammation is then a reaction, a healing process aimed at eliminating foreign substances or processes, and one must know how to respect it. It would be a grave error to combat it in all circumstances. It may happen that it constitutes in itself a danger through its intensity or localization, and in that case it is the duty of the doctor to moderate it, but to dispel it without due consideration would be to risk being engulfed in Scylla while avoiding Charybdis, and would expose the organism to no less a danger, albeit possibly at some later date.

Under the best conditions the end result of inflammatory processes is the regeneration of what has suffered injury, the reabsorption by the etheric body of what had become foreign. This is what takes place in healing by primary intention, for example.[1] But the matter is not always so simple. Foreign substances, those which in other words have become inaccessible to the human etheric forces, often constitute ideal nourishment for microorganisms, which settle and proliferate there. Infection is always a secondary process. We can certainly induce an experimental disease by the inoculation of a virus, but that has no more in common with current infections than a revolver shot has with a box on the ear. The defences of the organism are incited in a much more intense manner in infections than in simple inflammation, and we recognize therein the action of the ego through the other bodies. What was local heat here becomes *fever*. The formation of antibodies can also be considered as a manifestation of the ego, for these are a factor in the individualization of the blood. The astral body provokes, in addition to pain, elimination through the excretions. The leucocytic hyperactivity which results in pus formation is dependent on the etheric body.

When a child comes into the world he is still soft, his form is imprecise and his body consists of about 70% water (that of the adult still consisting of 60%). The skull bones are still elastic and incomplete, leaving membranous spaces between them which are the fontanelles. Little by little the child's structures become firmer. Not only his bones but also his skin, and in fact all his tissues, harden, and this process continues till death. This hardening is accompanied by a progressive diminution in the tendency to inflammations.

If we relate these facts to statements in Chapter 4, we have to admit that the action of the ego at the superior pole is, in the end, more marked than at the inferior pole and that the nerve-sense processes take precedence over those of metabolism. If we call to mind that the ego and the astral body detach themselves from the superior pole during sleep, the metabolic functions then becoming more active, this fact does not surprise us any longer. In fact we sleep on average eight hours and are awake for sixteen. While we are awake, nerve-sense processes predominate, with their natural consequences of tissue breakdown and mineralization. What has been destroyed during the day is not completely regenerated during the night, which explains why, in the long run, the organism is damaged and grows old—in a word becomes sclerotic. Up to a certain point these processes are normal, but beyond this they become pathological.

In the hardening and mineralization of the body, and in the build-up of mineral deposits accompanying this, we have a process directly opposite in character to inflammation, which tends towards dissolution. These two processes often alternate in man. If inflammation is the reaction to mineralization and to hardening, sclerosis on the other hand is often a reaction to a process of dissolution. This is shown for example in cicatrization, where a stage of consolidation appears after an inflammatory stage. Doctors often observe particularly rapid processes of sclerosis and ageing following inflammatory conditions. This is seen in a striking manner in many old cases of tuberculosis. We also see patients of a plethoric-digestive, and consequently inflammatory, type later develop particularly rapid and intense sclerosis. This law of the swing of the pendulum aids us in understanding these apparently paradoxical symptoms.

The treatment of inflammation consists particularly in aiding rather than hindering the organism in its own attempts at healing. We employ two basic remedies for this purpose: *Apis* and *Belladonna*. A bee sting (*Apis*) is accompanied by the four symptoms—calor, dolor, tumor and rubor—of inflammation. This constitutes in itself an indication for its use from the homoeopathic point of view without, however, explaining the process of healing. We cannot understand the action of *Apis* without considering the hive in its entirety, which represents a whole organism in itself.[2] This organism possesses a peculiarity unique in the world of insects—that of creating a uniform temperature which is approximately the same as human blood. A characteristic such as this gives us an idea of the connection between the hive and the ego. By the administration of *Apis* we introduce into the organism heat processes similar to those which manifest in inflammation under the influence of the ego. We provoke, in a sense, an artificial inflammation which substitutes itself for the disease condition, thereby helping the organism to defend itself. Another characteristic of the hive is the hexagonal structure of the cells, reminiscent of the crystal forms of the mineral kingdom. There appears to be a true polarity between the almost human temperature of the environment in the hive and the mineral-like structure of the cells. It is this polarity, similar to the polarity between the mineralizing action of the ego at the upper pole and its heat action at the lower pole of man, which points the way to the therapeutic use of *Apis*.

In order to understand the action of *Belladonna*, it is necessary to picture to oneself this plant in its natural environment: the damp half-shade of the undergrowth. Its rapid growth in spring is the expression of intense etheric forces; then, on the appearance of its first flower, this outburst of growth is abruptly brought to a halt, giving the impression that other forces have thwarted the growth.

We have seen that, as a general principle, plants possess a physical body and an etheric body only. At the level of the roots the mineral forces are predominant, while at the level of the leaves the etheric forces are most important. With the flower the plant approaches the animal kingdom, just 'touching into' astral forces though these remain outside it. Such is the situation in the 'normal' plant, but in the poisonous plants this astrality penetrates into them, instead of remaining outside them, and expresses itself on the physical plane by the production of toxic substances. That is why *Belladonna* seems as though thwarted in its growth. These astral forces are in opposition to the etheric forces, restraining them in the same way as we have observed in the animal. If such plants are eaten, a foreign astrality with which it is unable to cope is introduced into the organism. Such is the process of intoxication.

The presence of astral forces within a plant tends to confer on it qualities that are characteristic of animals. So that we can say that in *Belladonna* there appears a desire—and a desire is a typical astral manifestation—to open up itself to the outside world and particularly to the light. But the plant does not possess organs which permit it to see. It would like to open wide the eyes which it does not possess. It can do this only inside an animal or human organism and therefore causes dilation of the pupils, and the eye reacts as if it were in darkness.

Another astral manifestation of desire is compulsive movement which also appears as restlessness in cases of poisoning by *Belladonna*.

We find this conflict between the etheric and astral once

again in another group of symptoms of Belladonna poisoning: the flushed face, headache and throbbing pulse. These reflect resistance to the opposite process, to the direct action of the astral body on the physical body. What, in the case of *Apis*, occurs between the ego and the physical body, in the case of *Belladonna* occurs between the astral body and the etheric body. We help the body to re-establish equilibrium by giving *Belladonna* in a dilute form.

The mixture *Apis* 3x/*Belladonna* 3x aa is thus the basic treatment in inflammatory conditions, especially when they affect the respiratory passages. In infections of the throat we give it in the form of *Bolus eucalypti* comp., by pharyngeal insufflation, alternately with *Mercurius cyanatus* 4x, every one to two hours. One has to be very courageous the first time one uses such a treatment in place of serum in a case of diphtheria, but the results are so conclusive that I doubt if anyone who has once tried this treatment would ever go back to the use of serum.

In cases of erysipelas, abscesses and furunculosis we give *Carbo betulae* 5%/*Sulphur* 1% in addition to *Apis* 3x/*Belladonna* 3x hourly alternately with the latter.

It is necessary to control the inflammation when it threatens to be dangerous in itself. In the case of high temperatures we consider compresses, packs and, especially, baths given at a temperature 2°C below that of the patient (do not forget to precede this with a mild cardiac tonic or, better, by five to ten drops of Cardiodoron—*Primula*/*Onopordon*/*Hyoscyamus*). On being taken out of the bath the patient is wrapped up in a bath towel without being dried. He is then put to bed once more and given an infusion of elder or lime blossom to drink in order to stimulate perspiration. This at the same time assists in lowering the temperature and also helps the organism to get rid of toxins. In this way we facilitate the displacement of the disease to the periphery (cf. the use of mustard plasters, p. 83) and this will make it easier to cure.

If the temperature continues we give an injection of *Argentum* 20x or 30x every two or three days. This remedy is not intended to combat the fever itself but the harmful effects which its persistence can entail.

Is it possible to abandon the use of antibiotics? The important thing is, in fact, not to condemn one remedy and to extol another in its place, but to be fully conscious of what one is doing. We have seen that microorganisms are agents, not causes, of disease. It does not then seem logical to direct our attack primarily at them, for this would be the equivalent merely of dispelling one of the symptoms and in short of masking or metamorphosing the illness, which would manifest itself again sooner or later on another plane. One becomes well aware of this when one compares two patients treated for the same condition, the first by antibiotics and the second by simply helping the organism to defend itself. The first drags on often for months, is unable to recover his strength and gives the impression of not being himself. The second, on the contrary, after a 'sharp' illness, gives the impression both mentally and physically of regeneration and renewal. He declares, if he has been well cared for, that he feels *better* than before his illness. The patient treated with antibiotics may in contrast resemble a person who, instead of paying a debt, contracts a new loan which is even heavier to bear. The inefficacy of a treatment can often be due to a previous treatment with antibiotics. In such a case it is recommended that one should start by prescribing a dose of *Penicillium* in a potency of 5th, 7th or 9th, the higher potency if a long time has elapsed since administering the antibiotic. It should be recognized that the repeated use of antibiotics, apart from their well-known disadvantages, also weakens the development of inflammatory reactions by the organism, thus making a nidus for cancer to develop.

If childhood is the age of inflammation, old age on the other hand tends towards sclerosis. But not all elderly people are its victims, and we see it appear also in relatively young subjects. Sclerosis is then a morbid process only in so far as it is an exaggeration of the normal process of hardening. Before discussing treatment of it, one might well consider if prophylaxis against this condition is possible. Such treatment must be derived from our studies of the origin of this process. Everything that exaggerates the direct action of the ego on the physical body will favour sclerosis, particularly in early childhood, for acceleration of the process of hardening in a young person will continue for the rest of his life. It is therefore not paradoxical to say that the prevention of this condition should start at birth. We will talk of this again when studying the child. When sclerosis is established it is already more difficult to combat it, and it is as well to start its treatment from the very first signs. We employ two principal remedies for this, birch and lead.

If we observe a birch tree when its leaves have only just unfolded in the sunny spring air, we can ourselves experience that this tree is expressive of youth. In his first course of lectures for doctors, Rudolf Steiner shows us how certain particular characteristics of the birch are the reflection of an organic human process. He states that man resembles the animal in his most central functions, i.e. in the processes of digestion, of blood transformation and in respiration. In these, like the animal, he transforms vegetable proteins; and thus, in administering vegetable substances as medicines, we have to look especially to those central functions and call on the processes acting between the animal kingdom and the vegetable kingdom.

Rudolf Steiner tells us of an analogous action to the above

that takes place more towards the periphery 'between heaven and earth', between the ego, partaking of the cosmic, and the mineral world. Here, at the level of the skin, we can observe a process of salt elimination or demineralization. In administering a mineral remedy we call on the highest element in man, on his ego, which should be capable of overcoming this mineral and of destroying it. This is what happens when, for example, we administer silica.

We find something analogous to this in the birch: on the one hand a process of protein synthesis which is concentrated in the young leaves, and on the other hand an elimination of mineral salts, in this case of potassium, in the bark. Rudolf Steiner tells us that these are two separate processes in the birch; and that if they were intermingled the birch would be a magnificent herbaceous plant. This tendency to separation of the two processes is found in other trees, but it is especially marked in the birch. Its bark will therefore be a suitable remedy for stimulating this elimination of minerals from the skin in man. Therefore we prescribe it in sclerosis, and also in the dry dermatoses which give the impression that the skin is no longer capable of eliminating minerals correctly.

We employ the bark of the birch preferably by subcutaneous injection since we are aiming at the periphery, in the form of *Betula cortex* 1% to 2%, two to three subcutaneous injections a week.

In sclerosis, as in rheumatic infections, it is also of service to call on this central synthesizing process that we have described. We therefore give extracts of the young leaves by mouth. A particularly pleasant form of this remedy is Birch Elixir. We can also use the young leaves in an infusion.

This example of birch shows us in a particularly tangible way the connections and similarities that can exist between nature and man, an understanding of which leads us further on the therapeutic path.

We shall consider lead in more detail in a later study of the metals. We shall be content for the moment to indicate the form in which we prescribe it in sclerosis: *Plumbum mellitum* 12x trit. When sclerosis affects the cerebral region in particular we can also give it as 20x. These triturations should be given two or three times a day, a quarter of an hour before meals, in a teaspoonful of Birch Elixir. It is as well to make a break after four to six weeks, during which one prescribes *Argentum* 6x which will correct any excessive action brought about by the lead treatment.

Part Two

THE STAGES OF HUMAN DEVELOPMENT

In the first part of this book we attempted to develop a new view of the human being. We considered man as composed of four constituent elements. These are present in differing ways in the three structural and functional divisions of man; that is, in the nerve-sense pole, the rhythmic system and the metabolic pole. The relationship between these two aspects of man changes during the course of his growth and development.

In the second part of our study we shall review these developmental changes in seven-year periods.

It might seem to the reader that we devote too large a space in these chapters to the education of the child. We believe, however, that education has an enormous influence on health throughout a person's life, and that this influence is one we cannot ignore.

FROM BIRTH TO THE AGE OF SEVEN

If the adult human is the most highly evolved being in creation, at birth in contrast he is less advanced in his development than any other creature. This is not surprising, for the richness and variety of his faculties necessitate long maturation and the maintaining of a plasticity that allows progressive remodelling of his structures.

The animal is essentially in possession of all its faculties from the time of birth. After birth they are brought to greater perfection but there is no acquisition of new faculties. The faculties it possess are highly specialized and are brought to a much greater degree of perfection than in man. Thus the claw of the cat is much better adapted to a certain mode of hunting than the human hand, but the potential of the claw for other activities is extremely limited.

In contrast the hand of man is capable of carrying out an infinite number of tasks but each has to be learned. To what perfection can it not attain! Think of the hand of the sculptor, of the watchmaker or of the pianist. However, this learning activity is only possible with the help of other human beings. An animal, in contrast, is able to do things by instinct. A duck, even if hatched by a hen or in an incubator, swims without having to be taught.

The development of the human being takes place roughly in periods of seven years, of which the milestones or land-marks are the second dentition and puberty. It is interesting to note that this rhythm corresponds to the seven-year period taken for a total renewal of the physical substance of our bodies. At birth the human being is the result of hereditary components received from the parents. On this stream of heredity, by which we belong to a race, a people and a family, is superimposed what we bring of our own, which will make us an individual unlike any other. This constitutes the indestructible spiritual kernel of our being which unites itself with our earthly body at each incarnation. It also enters and leaves the body in waking and sleeping. Considered in purely material ways, the human being remains totally incomprehensible. If man were nothing but the result of heredity there would be no greater difference between two human beings than there is between two sheep.

What man brings from the spiritual world comes into opposition with the hereditary stream throughout the first seven years of life and leads to the creation of a physical body that is both compatible with the structure of our ego and also a suitable instrument for its expression. If we observe the evolution of a child attentively, we will understand that heredity and environment are insufficient to explain it.

If we look at a baby, we are struck by the relative size of its head. The rest of the body, and the limbs particularly, appear almost to be appendages to the head. The earlier in the development of the embryo one looks, the more evident is this relative importance of the cephalic pole. The fertilized ovum can really be considered as being originally nothing more than a head.

Despite this large head the child is unable to think. Is that to say that the head is inactive? As before, it is Rudolf Steiner who gives us the key to this enigma. It is from the head, he says, that the growth forces arise which model the rest of the body, and until the body has reached a certain degree of development these forces are not available for thinking.

These growth forces are in fact etheric forces, which manifest themselves in the rhythmic, repetitive manner seen in the phenomenon of cellular multiplication and also in the desire to imitate, a characteristic of the child during its first seven years—for imitation is also a process of *reproduction*. The child has a compelling need to imitate and for this reason the example given by the parents and, in a more general way, by all the people who come into contact with the child has a major importance not only for the child's moral development but also for the proper formation of his physical organism. In repeating what he sees done the child truly has an effect on the development of his physical body. This is as true for good influences as for bad. Thus whether harmony prevails or not in the child's surroundings has profound repercussions on his whole being. As development proceeds, the etheric forces take on other tasks, and their connections with other elements of the human being change, so that it will not be possible to make up for anything that has been neglected, nor to restore what has been deformed. We have a typical example of this in 'wolf-children'[1]—those children who have been brought up by an animal and have themselves becomes animals. In such cases no efforts at education can now succeed in making them into true human beings. N. Glas[2] has related a less tragic case in a quotation from E. S. Waterhouse's *Psychology and Pastoral Work* (London, 1939). It concerns a four-year-old child who was brought to the Tavistock Clinic because it was thought that he was insane, as he did not speak and spent his time running about barking like a dog. It was discovered on investigation that the child had been brought up by a nurse who merely left him in his play-pen, otherwise only cleaning and feeding him. The woman had several dogs to which she was greatly attached, and on which she lavished great affection. When an understanding and devoted person was found to look after him, the child developed rapidly and became normal over about eighteen months.

It would be quite mistaken to seek for any conscious intent on the part of the child in this situation, or to think that there was any method in his strange behaviour. We see here the primal need to imitate which is characteristic of that age. It is not at all surprising that this need to imitate manifested in imitation of the dogs, rather than towards the nurse from whom he received no affection. We could even say that the child had also imitated the nurse in her indifference towards him, another human being. He himself became indifferent towards her.

This example makes us more conscious of the extreme importance that Rudolf Steiner attributed to the example given by adults to children in the first seven-year period. He summarized this in the words: 'To educate a child is to educate yourself.' It is not only the circle of people around a child that is important but the whole environment in which he finds himself. Ugly surroundings in poor taste, crude colours, mechanical music or, even worse, television, are effectively poisons or even physical traumas which leave an indelible imprint on the physical body of the child. The case of the Tavistock Clinic child also helps us to understand why Rudolf Steiner advised against giving children toys with the shape of animals before they could walk. Generally speaking, toys have a considerable influence on the development of the child. Those which are a mere caricature of the living world should not be used, nor those with a too lifelike appearance which leaves no room for the child's imagination. The younger a child the greater is the importance of the environment, and so harmonious surroundings should be created from the time of birth. The cold, impersonal atmosphere of some maternity wards is indisputably just the opposite of what one would wish for. For the sake of convenience—what errors this leads us into—the newborn baby can be isolated from his mother when his right place is at her side. He needs the warmth of his mother— not only the physical warmth but the spiritual warmth of a mother's love. Since it is impossible to demonstrate this with the help of a thermometer, it is merely declared that it does not exist or that it is of no importance! It will one day be realized that the arbitrarily instituted measures of our day arising from our ignorance of true human nature have their repercussions, not only on people's mental state but also on physical health, giving rise to conditions manifesting even in old age. Here is an example. From time immemorial mothers have rocked their children, knowing instinctively that it was good for them. But one day a pedant decreed that this caused a bad habit in the child, and the whole world hastened to repeat this dogma; for the authority of 'experts' has never flourished before so much as it does in our time. Yet American researchers who interrogated adults to find out if they had been rocked as babies discovered that those who had been rocked later led a happier and more harmonious existence. When a child is rocked his rhythmic activity is nourished and his emotional life is harmonized. The same line of thought supports the custom of singing lullabies to children and the idea that later they should be told fairy tales such as the excellent ones by the brothers Grimm and by de Perrault.

The environment and the emotional contact are a part of what the child receives from the external world. Food is another part, and its influence on development is no less important. In the first six months of life, anything other than the milk of the mother should only be a last resort. As Dr R. Leroi has said: 'The breast, at first an expression of female beauty, has to metamorphose into an organ of benevolence which proffers itself.' The desire to preserve this beauty to the detriment of the health of the child is a manifestation of egoism which can expose a woman later to the danger of cancer of the breast. People are not sufficiently aware that half the women who suffer from cancer of the breast have

never suckled a child and in the other half the majority of
women have had fewer than three children and have only
suckled for a short period.[3] One is sometimes surprised that
many mothers resort to the feeding-bottle when breast-
feeding is so simple, and one can well imagine that commer-
cial propaganda for dried and preserved milks may have
something to do with this fashion.

It is, moreover, false to claim that the deformation of the
breast is an inevitable consequence of breast-feeding.

We can get an idea of the importance of breast-feeding by
comparing growth of offspring and composition of milk in
man and three mammals in the graph below:

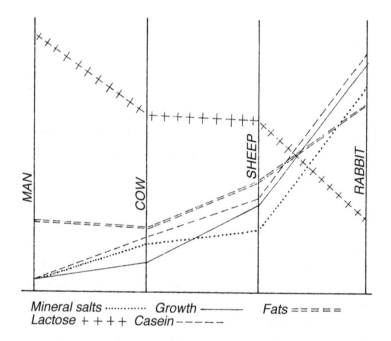

Mineral salts ············ Growth ——————   Fats = = = = =
Lactose + + + + Casein — — — — —

We see that the rate of growth is practically proportional to
the level of casein and mineral salts (CaO + MgO + P_2O_5).
The level of fats also follows the same curve but not so

closely. The level of lactose, on the contrary, is inversely proportional to the rate of growth. Naturally, cow's milk given to an infant will not make him grow three times as fast, but it nevertheless causes an increased retention of mineral salts in the proportion of 2.30 g. to 1.45 g., compared with breast milk, for an increase of weight of 100 g. Artificial feeding then leads to a more rapid mineralization. It is easy to observe that this is accompanied by a more rapid awakening of consciousness. Artificial feeding therefore brings about acceleration of development and consequently a premature ageing.

We have seen that in order to be assimilated, foodstuffs must be first broken down. An infant's powers of digestion are very limited as the forces necessary for this are not yet available. That is why he is so subject to alimentary disturbances. It is therefore important not to overpower the digestive forces by offering unsuitable food and to make changes of food gradually.

Certain paediatricians have recommended that meat should be given to children very early, for they have shown its influence on the development of muscles. This is undeniable, but is it desirable? It should be understood that if we accelerate the child's development by giving meat, then its development will cease that much earlier in proportion to the degree of acceleration, and for this reason will very likely remain incomplete. The reason that so many adults today retain a childlike mentality throughout their lives is certainly connected with the way they were fed as children. Let us recall again that eggs given prematurely to a child often cause him to lose his natural instinct to choose the right foods. In addition, owing to their sex hormone content, giving too many eggs may cause premature puberty, another undesirable form of growth acceleration.

A detailed description of the children's nutrition is beyond the scope of this book. More specialized works, such as those of Dr W. zur Linden[4] and Dr N. Glas,[5] are highly recommended.

The forces which work to form the rest of the organism arise in the cephalic pole, which is physically the most developed, while at the digestive and motor pole, which is still in a relatively undeveloped state, are found particularly intense will forces, an expression of the ego which models this organism from outside to make it its instrument. We find these will forces again in the processes of nutrition and they are expressed by the fervour with which an infant takes his mother's breast. We can notice how the whole body from the lips to the toes takes part in this activity. This will shows itself equally in the infant's crying and in all his liveliness, which contrasts with the feeble development of his limbs.

The child's movements, which at first seemed quite confused, gradually become purposeful. He starts by lifting his head, then tries to raise his body and soon succeeds in sitting up. Finally, after immense efforts, he stands upright and learns to walk. The fact of arriving at standing upright on both legs is a culmination of an untiring repetition of attempts and the exertion of a will force of which we can form an idea only with difficulty, and of which very few adults would be capable. Only those who have sought perfection in some form of activity, in playing a musical instrument for example, can have an idea of this. If one is at first astonished that anthroposophy connects the will with the pole of movement, observation of a child learning to walk will teach us how much this connection is justified. The child learns to speak almost at the same time. As in the case of walking, the child acquires speech by imitation. This faculty is intimately bound up with respiration and thus represents an affective manifestation. But, especially at first, speech is above all movement, use of the lips, and thus voluntary activity. It is only later, as a rule when he is able to walk, that the child starts to think, that is to say to grasp the relation between the sound which he produces and its meaning. Walking, talking and thinking are three great victories won by the child over an organism of which he has acquired a certain mastery. There are no comparable achievements in the animal, for it gambols around naturally without any particular effort of learning being necessary. The ability to stand on its feet is given to it and does not have to be acquired.

The appearance of the first teeth more or less coincides with learning to walk. Their eruption is also a manifestation of inner will. It is frequently accompanied by inflammatory processes and fever. The hardness of the tooth may make us think of a foreign body which the organism is trying to expel by inflammation. This does not, of course, go as far as total expulsion, but the hardest part, the enamel, is extruded to the exterior. If the tooth has too great difficulty in coming through, the will forces, thwarted in their endeavour, may react back into the organism and express themselves in cramps and convulsions.

The child has learnt to make his feelings and wishes clear in words by about three years old and then begins to distinguish himself from the outside world with which he had till then been intimately mingled. He no longer calls himself by his first name, as if he were an external object for himself like any other object, but he says 'I'. His spiritual being, his ego, has incarnated more deeply as his physical body forms and becomes more fitted to receive it. At the same time he becomes conscious of the outer world, distinguishing this from his inner being, which becomes stocked with memories. This taking hold of consciousness is generally accompanied by a need for self-assertion which shows itself by a tendency to say 'No' to everything suggested to him. This is very irritating for the parents but usually passes the more quickly the less it is opposed. As before, the child continues to imitate those around him, but now does so in a more conscious manner. The imitation had up to this time had a rather instinctive character, but now the child really wants to do things like his mother or father, preferably without help. It is necessary that this need to imitate should be allowed to develop freely. If it is opposed in the child, it will have a tendency to manifest again much later, possibly making him a mere imitator of others in adult life. It is possible that if children were allowed to satisfy their need to imitate more fully, they would not become slaves of all kinds of fashions when they become adults. It is certainly not possible to allow a child to do whatever he wants, and a wealth of imagination and great presence of mind are needed to succeed in the gentle guidance of a child. Education is truly an art!

With the shedding of his milk teeth at the end of the first seven-year period the child will have entirely renewed his physical substance. He will have built himself a body that is truly his own, whose proportions approximate more to those of an adult than those of a newborn child. The relationship between his head and his limbs has become such that the child can, by passing one arm over his head, reach the ear of the opposite side, and this is an excellent test of his mental maturity and readiness for school. We shall see why a little later on.

The intense work of developing his body gives rise to a lowered resistance to illness in the child before the age of seven years. He has inadequate powers of defence against external influences and it is therefore necessary to make sure that he is properly nourished as a protection against these external attacks. Exposure to noise, cold, heat or too intense light can give rise to disturbances. Temperature regulation, which is dependent on the ego, is not fully competent as long as the latter has not taken firm possession of the body, so that full self-regulation of temperature appears only gradually. Whereas light which is too strong can become a cause of suffering or illness for a small child, a lack of light, although this is much rarer now than it was a century ago, can result in rickets.

This condition is a typical expression of disequilibrium between the growth forces and the form-giving forces of the organism, and it merits further consideration.

Study of a rachitic bone shows us on the one hand an inadequate calcification, indicating a disturbance of metabolism, and on the other hand utterly confused proliferation of the connective tissue of the bone. We are thus confronted with both inadequate mineralization and lack of formative force. These two processes are, as we have already seen, carried out by the direct action of the ego on the organism. In rickets, the ego is too weak to carry out these processes or to ensure the metabolism of light and its integration with the chemical activity of the bones. It can also happen that the ego has not enough light at its disposal, but this exogenous form of rickets is now rare.

It is customary to give infants synthetic vitamin D for the prevention or treatment of rickets. This practice is not very satisfactory from the therapeutic point of view and is not without danger. It provides only a substitute for a natural substance rather than aiming at the root of the trouble. In the first place, while vitamin D acts on mineralization, it has in contrast no form-giving effect and so there is a risk of fixing the illness instead of healing it. Secondly, it may cause complications of hypercalcification, particularly in the kidneys, which are sometimes fatal. Even if such grave complications are relatively rare, the systematic administration of vitamin D nevertheless entails a premature hardening, not only of the bones but of all the tissues. It is not uncommon to see children who have been given this vitamin looking like little old men

and women with heads that are too small and whose sub-
sequent development cannot proceed normally. We shall
again come across this tendency to hurry treatment, which is
one of the evils of our time.

In a condition connected with the forces of light and the
ego, we think in the first place of *Phosphorus* given in 5x or 6x
strength, three drops before breakfast and before the midday
meal. (*Phosphorus* must never be given in low dilution in the
evening.) If the illness especially affects the cephalic pole
(craniotabes), *Phosphorus* 30x, five drops *every two or three
days*, is given at about 6 p.m. *Quartz* 10x trit. is given to
stimulate the form-giving forces. In the case of bone
deformities *Stannum* 10x trit. is prescribed, a saltspoonful
twice a day. *Stannum* is also used in cases of craniotabes in the
form of an ointment (*Stannum* 0.1% ungt.) for inunction of
the whole head at night. *Ferrum meteoricum* 20x, a saltspoonful, is given on waking to strengthen the ego's wish to
stand upright.

For the prevention of rickets it is a good thing to give the
mother during her pregnancy Calcium Supplements nos. 1
and 2 (no. 1: *Apatite* 6x/*Curcubita* 3x in the morning and
no. 2: *Conchae vera* 5%/*Quercus robur* 3x in the evening).
These are likewise given to the child from the ninth week
onwards.

It is good to train oneself to recognize if children belong to
the type with a large or with a small head. The metabolic
system predominates in the large-headed, and they have a
tendency to slower calcification. In the latter, the small-
headed, hardening is more rapid. Consequently in the former
only Calcium Supplement no. 2 is prescribed, and starting
later. Eventually it will be replaced by *Conchae* 3x to 6x. It is
good practice to continue the Calcium Supplements
throughout childhood up till the approach of puberty. They
are given for periods of four weeks followed by one or two

weeks' break. They are not given between 15 June and 15 September.[6] Calcium Supplements are not always sufficient as an adequate prophylaxis against rickets. If necessary, five drops of *Phosphorus* 6x on waking are given in addition during the period of the year when sunlight is deficient.

For the treatment of conditions due to hypervitaminosis D, *Argentum sulphur. nat.* 6x trit., a saltspoonful two or three times a day is given. This should be replaced if necessary by *Argentum* 6x trit. in fair children who are too sensitive to sulphur. Warm sulphur baths can also be given (one teaspoonful of *Kalium sulph.* 30% to the bath).

The diseases of childhood are acute manifestations of the struggle between the ego and the forces of heredity. At times the spiritual being may work particularly strongly on the physical body. This endeavour to rebuild and individualize the physical body gives rise to a predisposition to scarlet fever. At other times the spiritual being is more unstable and tends to give way to the earthly model. The child will then be susceptible to measles. This condition gives one the impression of a watery illness: the eyes water and the eyelids swell, and there is a somewhat puffy appearance of the whole body. These symptoms are manifestations of the etheric which we know has the body fluids as its supportive element. In contrast, scarlet fever, with its more dramatic character, makes one think of a conflagration. The dryness of the skin and the sandy feel of the rash recall the mineralizing action of the ego whose fire leaves ashes. This mineralizing action is found also in the complications of scarlet fever, which are nephritis and rheumatism.

The treatment of measles is straightforward. The child is given Infludo (or *Ferrum phos.* comp.), three to six drops according to age every two hours, and a mustard plaster is applied once daily to the chest to help the rash to come out. If the rash comes out well there is less risk of complications. The child must be kept warm and quiet for an adequate period and a fluid diet is prescribed while he is febrile. When the temperature begins to come down, Infludo is given less frequently, but should not be stopped abruptly. When necessary Weleda Cough Elixir is given (never any codeine mixture) or, better, an infusion of Sytra Tea with a little honey added. As well as being very efficacious, this is free from toxic effects. During convalescence *Ferrum meteoricum* 10x is given, a saltspoonful once or twice daily, and three teaspoonfuls of Sandthorn Elixir daily.

In scarlet fever it is best to treat the pharynx in the first place by applying a powder of *Bolus eucalypti* comp. every four hours. If the throat is red *Cinnabar* 20x in a saltspoonful is also given every four hours (two hours after each application of the powder). If there is a marked exudate on the tonsils or pharynx, *Cinnabar* is replaced by *Mercurius cyanatus* 4x, five to ten drops according to age. The basic treatment for scarlet fever is *Cassiterite* 0.1% trit., one dessertspoonful of which is added to a bath at a temperature 2°C below that of the patient. One should not forget to give a cardiac tonic (five to ten drops of Cardiodoron) before the bath. If a bath is not possible, it is replaced by a cold compress round the whole body, a towel being moistened with cold water and sprinkled with a dessertspoonful of *Cassiterite*. After the bath or cold compress the patient is rolled up in a dry bath towel and given an infusion of elder or lime flowers to provoke sweating. The bath or compress is given once a day unless a high temperature necessitates a greater frequency. The heart should always be supported by giving Cardiodoron at least three times a day in a dose of five or ten drops. As in all acute febrile illnesses a liquid diet should be prescribed and great caution should be employed in returning to a fuller diet, in particular salt and protein are excluded. During convalescence *Ferrum meteoricum* 10x,

Pancreas 6x aa trit. and *Equisetum* 6x dil. are given even in the absence of signs of nephritis. If it is treated in this way there is little risk of complications from scarlet fever.

If scarlet fever makes us think of the element fire and measles of the element water, whooping cough unquestionably corresponds to the element air and the astral body. It is characterized particularly by the fits of coughing which are familiar to all of us, and which represent a desperate attempt by the organism to get rid of the air contained in the lungs. In normal respiration the union between the astral body and the physical organism varies in a rhythmic manner, but in whooping cough, as a result of the irritation of the bronchi, the astral forces remain fixed firmly to the body, causing spasm of the glottis and retention of the air. The trapped air then acts as a foreign body which the organism tries to expel, but this is impossible because of the closure of the glottis.

Finally the increasing carbon dioxide content of the blood gives rise to a tendency to syncope and therefore to a detachment of the astral body. The spasm gives way and the air enters the lung again with a whistling sound. It may seem a paradox that a desperate attempt to expel air ends in an inspiration. In reality it is the residual air which acts as a foreign body which the organism tries to expel; and on the opening of the glottis the air penetrates by the mere elasticity of the thorax. If you observe a child during a spasm, you will see that, as Dr Steiner said, it is a matter of expiratory dyspnoea, and you will have a lively understanding of the behaviour of the astral body.

The part played by the astral body makes one understand the importance of the emotional factor in whooping cough. Children of anxious mothers suffer from this condition more severely and dramatically than those whose mothers keep calm. The following is a typical example of this. I had been treating a child with whooping cough shortly before going on a journey and had handed him over to the care of a colleague the evening before my departure. Everything went off very well up to the moment when the mother learnt of my departure. Her anxiety had immediate repercussions on the child whose fits of coughing increased considerably in frequency and intensity, although the treatment had in no way been changed.

Therefore in order to treat a case of whooping cough one should start off by reassuring those in contact with the child and insist on a discipline which is in certain respects very strict. Above all the food intake must be considerably reduced. It is not always easy to achieve this, for a mother is always afraid of her child dying of hunger but never of dying from overeating! When there is vomiting a light meal is given after a fit of coughing. If vomiting is frequent, one should think of compensating for the loss of chlorides by giving salt. There is a danger of rapid dehydration caused by vomiting in an infant, and one must be alert to counteract this and only give him milk much diluted with water or an infusion. One must also be very strict with regard to sedatives for the cough, for these are themselves the cause of many complications. Treatment aims at moderating the action of the astral body by means of Pertudoron 1 and 2. Excellent results are obtained provided that the dosage below is adhered to and the temptation to exceed this is resisted. An infant is given a maximum of three drops and an older child or adult not more than five. No. 1 and no. 2 are given alternately every two hours, each medicine thus being given four-hourly. At first the medicine is also given during the night. During the first day or two a slight aggravation of symptoms is generally noted *which must on no account lead to an increase in the dosage of the medicine or the frequency with which it is given*, but rather to their diminution. Then the condition improves. Setbacks are frequently due to overloading of the stomach.

One must not be afraid to see a child lose weight, for when the illness is over the child will show an excellent appetite and quickly regain his weight (unless the fits of coughing have been suppressed with codeine or its derivatives). Pertudoron is given until the total disappearance of the fits of coughing, but the frequency of its administration may be decreased when the child begins to improve. It is often possible to stop early with administration during the night.

It is interesting to note that after an attack of whooping cough a certain irritability of the bronchi sometimes continues to exist for more than a year, so that every time a child catches a cold his cough takes on to some extent the character of whooping cough.

If you observe a child treated in the above manner you will be surprised not only at the rapidity of the convalescence, but above all at the progress he will have made. This progress shows itself even in his speech. On the other hand a child in whom the illness has been repressed progresses very slowly for months and sometimes for years. Accordingly a child should never be vaccinated against whooping cough for this would deprive him of the possibility of development which is given to him by the illness.[7]

8

FROM SEVEN TO FOURTEEN YEARS
OF AGE

Up to the age of seven years the etheric body remains united with the maternal etheric in the same way as the physical body was united with that of the mother before birth. With the second dentition the etheric body in its turn becomes separate—in a sense, is born. Until this time it has been occupied in the growth and construction of the physical body and in remodelling its proportions. This activity we can see expressed in the changing proportion of the limbs to the head.

Part of the etheric body remains bound to the organism and continues to form the basis for processes of growth and regeneration. The other part, having accomplished its task on the physical plane, is set free. The question is, what functions does it now fulfil? For nothing in nature is ever lost and everything is metamorphosed. In this case those forces which have become free we find operating on the plane of thought, in memory, in the formation of mental images and in the linking-up of concepts. It is for the reasons we have stated that there is a certain dimensional relationship between the head and the limbs and that one can use this as an indication of mental maturity and readiness for formal schooling.

There is a marked similarity between the growth forces and those of thought, which is at first surprising. The table on the opposite page will give an idea of this.

For the etheric forces to become thought forces it is necessary that the ego should be sufficiently mature to be able to make use of them. It must take possession of them and bring them into order, otherwise they will tend to regress to

Action of the etheric body

On growth	On thought
Reproduction of organic elements, e.g. cells	Reproduction of thoughts (percepts) perceived in the mental image
Elaboration of symmetrical elements (right and left)	The ability to think of opposites
Plant structure	Thought structure
Variety of forms	Variety of thoughts
Concentration of growth potential in seeds	Memorizing (preservation of elements which can be recalled to consciousness)
Linking of one cell to another according to a plan	Linking of ideas in accordance with logic
Ramification, etc.	Association of ideas, etc.

the vegetative stage. Dyslexia is one expression of this regression. In this condition we find irregularities in the metamorphosis of the etheric body which manifest themselves on the plane of mental function in the form of mirror images or reversal of letters. These recall to us the faculty of symmetrical reproduction which is one of the properties of the etheric body. The child reads b in place of d, q in place of p, ne in place of en, cor in place of roc, etc. These disturbances are fortunately usually transitory and disappear completely when the ego succeeds in incarnating properly. We shall subsequently find another aspect of this regression of the etheric forces in connection with cancer.

Liberation of part of the etheric body makes possible the development of memory, so that it is at this age that the child becomes truly capable of learning. It is not impossible to teach a child to write from the age of three, but if this is done etheric forces are called upon prematurely which should be reserved for the building of the organism. Even if it does not entail immediate disturbances this premature utilization of forces will, sooner or later, have its repercussions on health, possibly even after seven years. The child will become pale and weak if we make too great a call on his memory and if too much is asked of the nerve-sense pole. If, on the other hand, too *little* is demanded, the blood processes of the metabolic pole will tend to prevail and the child will be excessively overflowing in spirits. It is easy to show that our present time usually makes too great a demand on the thought forces.

The partial liberation of the etheric body entails a greater freedom for the child with regard to his surroundings. That is a necessary condition for the development of the life of the emotions, a development which continues throughout the second seven-year period. This life of the soul is characterized by a perpetual fluctuation between two fundamental feelings to which we can attribute all that we feel—sympathy and antipathy (see note 3 to Chapter 1, p. 10). This fluctuation between two opposites is consequently a rhythmic alter-nation, and it is with the rhythmic system of the organism that we associate it. This system had been previously formed in the child, but does not develop fully, so as to become the instrument of the emotional life, until the period extending from the age of seven to fourteen. The formation of the organism is mainly under the direction of the etheric body up to the age of seven years, but from then onwards the astral body takes the lead. One may regard the emotions, the movements of the soul, as a kind of dance, sustained through sensory perceptions and expressed in the movement of the limbs. That is to say, there exists a fluctuation between the cephalic pole and that of mobility which produces a balance between them.

Before seven years of age the emotional life of the child is little developed and is primarily the expression of his relations with his physical surroundings. The child seeks the warmth of his mother, for example. He lives in his surroundings without really becoming conscious of the feelings of others and is surprisingly objective. He hardly experiences compassion and can show cruelty, because he lacks awareness of what others feel. When two small children play together, each largely plays for himself. It may be that one imitates the other, but there is little inner contact between them.

An interiorization of feeling which comes into relationship with the external world, appears when the astral body comes into play. Sympathies and antipathies are felt in the very depths of the soul. The child becomes capable of friendship, but also of enmity. He develops his social sense, he begins to play in a group, he can sing in unison or even in canon. Music plays a most important part in education at this period, for it helps to harmonize the forces of thinking and willing. It is not generally known that our body is constructed in harmony with the laws of music and in particular that the proportion of the different sections of the limbs is the same as that existing between musical intervals. We can therefore assist the development of the child by teaching him to play a musical instrument, and in general by all artistic activities. Education at this period should always have an artistic character and never become drily intellectual. School work will not then become a drudgery, and the child's natural curiosity will remain alert rather than being blunted by premature intellectuality.

An event occurs about the ninth year which reminds us of what happened between the second and third years—the process of incarnation of the ego. At that period it took possession of the nerve-sense pole; now it unites itself more strongly with the metabolic pole. It can happen that this process is hindered, and this can then cause metabolic disturbances, such as diabetes. Such diseases are an expression of an insufficient action of the ego on certain metabolic functions. It is interesting to note that diabetes makes its appearance more frequently at this age than at any other.

Apart from such problems as these, the second seven-year period of life is usually a time of good health because of the predominance of the rhythmic system, the harmonizer, during these years. For illness is always the expression of an excessive action of one of the poles which the rhythmic system endeavours to correct by re-establishing equilibrium.

Having united with the metabolic system at about the ninth year, the ego working from the central, rhythmic system gradually unites more closely with the muscles and bones. Movements, which previously had a more automatic character, now become more conscious, and this does not always happen without certain difficulties arising. One can see this for oneself by trying to carry out consciously some movement which one habitually makes without thinking. One may then recall to some small degree the awkwardness one felt when first learning a skill. When becoming more conscious of his limbs the child of about twelve years of age also becomes more awkward. He often does not know quite what to do with his arms and shoves his hands in his pockets; and when he takes them out he frequently drops things, to the great annoyance of those around him. This phase generally passes quite quickly, but it can happen that these disturbances are more severe, and then we have the condition of Chorea minor or St Vitus' Dance.

Let us recall what we said at the beginning about the astral body and its part in the interiorization of perceptions, and in the reaction to this which is exteriorization in the form of movements. There it is a question of true rhythm, of a 'respiration' in which the ego takes part in the bringing to consciousness of perceptions and in the voluntary expression that is movement. If the astral body is unable to fulfil its part, these processes will be carried out in a manner lacking rhythm; the ego will not be able to express itself harmoniously through the astral body and will then have difficulty in taking possession of the limbs. But the incapacity of the astral body to accomplish its task is the expression of a dominance of the etheric causing a certain 'viscosity', a certain inertia hindering the action of the astral body. We can now understand the symptoms of chorea. It often appears after stress, an emotional shock or a fright, which causes a weakening of the astral body. The first symptoms are respiratory disturbances. The appearance of involuntary movements could suggest an excessive activity of the astral body, but they are in reality the result of its fruitless attempts at becoming master of the situation. We can recall here the picture of the alpine climber (p. 54), which we evoked with regard to the subject of cramp, but with one fundamental difference. In cramp, movement freezes into rigidity and the processes of consciousness are painfully intensified. In chorea, movement is intensified in a chaotic manner and consciousness becomes blurred to extinction. This demonstrates that in cramps we have an excessively strong process arising from the nerve-sense pole (direct action of the ego and astral body on the organism) and in chorea an overly strong process arising from the pole of metabolism and movement (indirect action of the upper elements).

We can now readily understand why a similar condition can arise during pregnancy, which is also characterized by a dominance of the lower pole and of the etheric forces.

What is the treatment for chorea? In the first place the child is kept away from school to avoid the emotional trauma which his behaviour will arouse and which only aggravates his condition. One should consider arsenic, for Rudolf Steiner said: 'To give arsenic is to astralize.' But one must be careful with this remedy for one can easily overshoot the mark. It is preferable to use it in its natural combination with iron and copper, such as is found in certain mineral spa waters of northern Italy (Levico, Roncegno). It has never been possible to reproduce this natural combination in the laboratory. Iron helps the incarnation of the ego and copper harmonizes the action of the astral body. This mineral water can be prescribed in the form of *Levico* 3x, five drops to be taken in the morning and at midday. There is also an excellent remedy for chorea for which we are indebted to Dr Noll, one of the pioneers of anthroposophical medicine—Choreodoron 1 and 2. No. 1 is composed of *Agaricus* 4x/*Datura* 3x/*Mygale* 5x aa dil., and no. 2 of *Cuprum aceticum* 4x/*Zincum valerianum* 4x aa dil. No. 1 and no. 2 are given alternately every two hours in a dose of five drops. Sulphur baths (*Kalium sulphuratum* 30%, one teaspoonful to a hot bath) are also useful, for sulphur has the property of re-establishing the equilibrium between the astral body and the etheric body. Finally it is an excellent thing for the patient to do curative eurythmy if this is possible.

Chorea has sometimes been considered a complication of rheumatic fever. It often appears by itself, however. There is, nevertheless, a connection between these two conditions which have slightly different causes but entirely different symptoms. The etheric body has for its support all the body fluids which we call our 'water organism'. This has to be penetrated by a respiratory process, we could say 'ventilated' by the action of the astral body on our 'air organism'. This process of ventilation is inadequate in rheumatic fever and the respiratory function of the astral body is incomplete. The result of this is the appearance of what we can call 'etheric-aqueous residues', which behave like foreign bodies causing a predisposition to inflammatory and exudative reactions. Moreover it is people of a lymphatic temperament (especially those with a tendency to inflammations), i.e. those characterized by the predominance of the etheric and the water organism, who are the most liable to this disease. Dunbar[1] has noticed that these children have smooth faces and unconcerned expressions, giving them an angelic appearance. The way the illness travels from one joint to another gives us an impression of fluctuation as if this etheric residue, which escapes the action of the astral, was fleeing from it, and the astral body was not properly successful in assuming its function. As it is the metabolic processes which gain the upper hand, we can also understand why it is that the articulations of the neck, which have closer connections with the structure-building processes arising from the upper pole, are spared. We find the same thing with the small joints of the fingers, for we find equally at the periphery a predominance of the nerve-sense system over the metabolic which is primarily central. Moreover girls, who are less deeply incarnated, have a greater rheumatic tendency than boys. The abundant perspiration indicates the attempt of the astral body to overcome the water organism. Therefore sweating is a healthy process which it would be a mistake to oppose.

Our treatment, however, will attempt to stimulate the water organism. In the first place an infusion of *birch leaves* is given to encourage elimination and to help assimilation and metamorphosis of proteins. These will then have less tendency to be deposited in the form of exudates. It is also very important that the patient should, from the beginning of the illness, be put on a light vegetarian diet that is low in proteins and salt. As a basic remedy we prescribe five to ten drops every two hours of alternately Rheumadoron 1 and 2 (No. 1: *Aconitum nap. pl. tot.* 4x/*Arnica pl. tot.* 2x/*Bryonia rad.* 3x aa dil; No. 2: *Colchicum tuber. digest* 3x/*Juniperus sabina sumit.* 4x aa dil). Arnica 10% ointment is applied to the joints without rubbing, or barely damp arnica compresses are applied (one teaspoonful of arnica 20% in $\frac{1}{3}$ glass of water).

With this solution a piece of flannel is very lightly moistened—arnica and wool go well together—and applied to the
affected joint. It is remoistened once or twice a day and the
compresses are kept at the right temperature with the help of
a rubber hot-water bottle. The heart must not be forgotten,
and ten drops of Cardiodoron A should be given three times a
day. This treatment has always enabled me to obtain complete cures without complications and I have never had
recourse to salicylates and anti-inflammatory drugs.

Particular attention should be paid to rickets in the second
seven-year period, for this is the time when deformities such
as scoliosis, kyphosis and lordosis appear. These conditions
are rightly linked to sunlight, but have wrongly been attributed to mechanical causes such as prolonged sitting or
carrying school bags which are too heavy. We have seen that
the straightening up to the vertical and the upright position
are the result of the action of the ego. Animals have no ego
and are horizontal beings, even the monkeys. The ego, which
separates from the body during sleep, returns to it again in the
morning. This incarnation should normally take place
quickly and completely, manifesting in pleasure and animation. But subjected to the dry intellectual nature of our
education and to an overburdening of cerebral functions (it is
not the bag full of school books which is too heavy but the
head!) the ego only incarnates reluctantly and takes incomplete possession of the organism. The child wakes badly,
grumbles and drags himself around and his spine no longer
has the strength to resist gravity and becomes bent. Moreover
the etheric forces are monopolized by the intellectual processes to the detriment of the vegetative processes.

It is not possible to remedy such harmful effects by a mere
change in the curriculum—it is above all the manner of
teaching which has to be altered. From the medical point of
view one aims at strengthening the ego and the etheric body.

We first of all think of Calcium Supplements, of phosphorus (a dilution of 5x or 6x in the morning) and of iron (*Ferrum meteoricum* 10x). We can help the ego to take possession of the organism by rubbing the upper part of the back and shoulders with cold salt water on waking (one large handful of sea salt in two pints of water). *Prunus spinosa* 3x, ten drops three times a day, is given to strengthen the etheric body or, if possible, *Prunus spinosa c. ferro WALA*. In severe cases of Scheuermann's disease, removal from school must be considered, together with the administration of subcutaneous injections of *Disci comp. c. stanno* alternating with *Betonica* 3x/*Rosmarinum* 3x. Finally, curative eurythmy can also be of very great benefit here.

Throughtout the second seven-year period the action of the astral body on the organism brings about a profound transformation, a maturation culminating in puberty. What we notice externally, the general physical changes, the metamorphosis of the whole organism, takes place in a very short period in comparison with the inner activity that has been accomplished during the preceding seven years, and this makes them very striking. The pitch of the voice is lowered by an octave in the boy but by only a tone in the girl, showing that in her the process of incarnation is less deep than in the boy. The feminine form is also more rounded, an expression of the more intense action of the etheric forces. In the boy, on the other hand, the ego and the astral body take possession of the physical body more directly at the nerve-sense pole, and this is expressed by more angular forms, by an abdominal type of respiration (the astral body descends more deeply into the organism through the nerve-sense pole) and by a stronger tendency to intellectuality (predominance of the nerve-sense pole).

The astral body, having brought about these transformations, becomes free and available for other tasks. There happens to it what happened to the physical body on its arrival in the world and for the etheric body at the age of seven—we can say that the astral body is 'born' at about the age of fourteen.

This is generally considered to be a particularly difficult period. It is often an easier time for pupils of Rudolf Steiner schools, where the teaching methods employed take as much account of the realities of the soul and spirit as of those of the material world.

9

FROM FOURTEEN TO TWENTY-ONE YEARS OF AGE

The freeing of the astral body at about the age of fourteen years puts new forces at the disposal of adolescents which they have to learn to make use of. The way in which they do this gives us further evidence of the difference in the processes of incarnation in the two sexes. These astral forces in girls, who are less deeply incarnated than boys, show themselves in a more superficial manner, and are rather like a garment or like finery with which they can amuse themselves and can experiment to see what effect it will have on other people. They are often tempted to see just how far they can go, and a teacher needs much circumspection, presence of mind and also a good sense of humour. At this age there is no question of simply exercising authority as in the preceding seven-year period. At that time authority had its proper place, for it emanated from an indisputable superiority which the child can admire. After the age of fourteen, however, there is danger of the teacher's authority degenerating into authoritarianism which can easily arouse revolt.

In boys these free astral forces act more deeply, in a more inward manner, which often gives rise in them to a feeling of embarrassment, resulting in a tendency for them to retire into themselves and to become somewhat bearish, even to the extent of grunting by way of replying to people. Here authority will not help either. On the contrary, tact is needed, and discretion in showing a young man that the forces which he does not yet know how to employ will give him a heightened consciousness, a faculty of reasoning which he did not possess before. This is probably why interminable discussions between friends take place at this age.

In animals the peak of development is reached when the procreative function has developed, and it is this also which signifies the beginning of the decline into old age. By contrast, in man the curve of development continues to rise after puberty and even when the curve begins to descend on the physical level it can still continue to rise on the spiritual level right up to the time of death, provided that the individual does not surrender himself to material things and views.

We have, then, two possible ways in which the freed astral forces may be reintegrated, one masculine and the other feminine. If these possibilities develop to extremes, then certain morbid states develop. If this astrality is not controlled in the girl and she is incapable of using the astral forces under the control of her ego to structure the vital impetus of the ether forces, the astral forces will manifest mentally and emotionally in an erratic and uncontrolled way, and we may see hysteria develop, as discussed in Chapter 4. If, on the contrary, the masculine tendency is exaggerated, if the astral forces enter too deeply into the organism, the soul will be too much concerned with material things and especially with the body. This may manifest as a tendency to eroticism; over-preoccupation with the body can, in certain cases, even develop into schizophrenia. It is also of course possible for boys to be subject to hysteria and girls to eroticism or schizophrenia, but the opposite is nevertheless more frequent.

If this incarnation process fails to develop properly in girls, it can cause a condition which has become quite rare today: chlorosis. The practice of sports and the more intense life of our times generally compels the ego to take possession of the organism to some degree. In chlorosis the ego seems to hold itself aloof from the organism and only incarnates reluctantly, so that the patient has a feeling of being a stranger to the world. This failure of the incarnation processes shows itself on the physical plane as a hypochromic anaemia. The metabolism of iron, the metal of incarnation, cannot take place correctly without the forces of the ego. It is not a question of deficiency of iron, but of an inability of the organism to assimilate it properly, even when its administration in large doses affords a temporary relief to the disturbances that characterize this condition.

Therapy therefore seeks primarily to stimulate the metabolism of iron, and this is done by the use of the stinging nettle, *Urtica dioica*. This is one of the ingredients of Anaemodoron, the other being the strawberry plant, *Fragaria vesca*. The nettle acts less by the iron it contains than by the 'iron process' which characterizes it. The strawberry, we can say, directs this process towards the blood. We can also make use of *Ferrum per Urticam* 0.1%, or even 1%, in which the iron has undergone a process of dynamization by means of the plant (see note 7 to Chapter 4). Anaemia having a connection with light and the ego, we think of course of *Phosphorus* (6x in the morning) as we do in all conditions where there is a deficient process of incarnation. Finally we can give lead in 6x or 10x, but with caution, to girls who give the impression of just floating over the ground. Let us not forget copper, for it makes the organism receptive to iron. We shall use it once again in the form of an ointment (*Ungt. Cupri* 0.4%) by daily inunction in the splenic region. Before finishing with chlorosis let us recall that iron has as 'brothers' elements 27 and 28 in the periodic classification, one of which, cobalt, can be useful in persistent cases.

Although not belonging exclusively to the third seven-year period, tuberculosis frequently makes its appearance during this time. So that it is not out of place to speak of it here, particularly as it shows an aetiological relationship with hysteria. The latter we have characterized as an excess of the vegetative processes of synthesis and elaboration. When these overflow in the pulmonary region they create a disposition to tuberculosis there. Infection is thus not the beginning of the illness but is only the consequence of persistently abnormal conditions already present in the organism. This does not mean that infection does not occur, only that it shows itself less on the physical than on the mental plane. People who live together, apart from the possibility of a similar constitution where heredity comes into play, have a tendency to 'merge' into each other, and mimetic phenomena appear especially in those with a less strong ego, giving rise to similar morbid predispositions. The 'hysterical' type, with its great instability, is obviously especially exposed to this kind of infection. These ideas are supported by the well-known psychological characteristics found in the tuberculous. Such people are characterized by a lively imagination and an artistic sense, which are the opposite of the abstract thought arising from the form-giving forces of the nerve-sense pole. One often finds a certain lack of concern in these patients towards their physical condition which can even go so far as to become a flight from material reality, an expression of a real refusal to incarnate. This resembles what we described in the case of chlorotic anaemia.

Why should tuberculosis have this predilection for the lung? There is an interesting parallel between this fact and the low silica content of this organ. Of all the organs in the body the lung contains the least silica. The pancreas, the organ richest in silica, is on the other hand almost never affected. The suprarenal gland, another organ which is poor in silica, is another site chosen by the tuberculosis bacillus. These facts are even more striking when one knows that the right lung, which is the poorer of the two in silica, is more frequently attacked than the left.

Silica, or rock crystal, can be regarded as an expression of the form-giving forces of the upper pole. This is expressed in the metaphor 'the light of thought', referring to clear thought reaching to the point of abstraction. This type of thought is exactly what one does not find in tuberculosis patients. Tuberculosis is characterized by the appearance of vegetative processes, by the formation of exudates, caseous material and pus. These last are an expression of the forces of metabolism. After tuberculosis is healed, it is the processes that are opposed to mineralization and calcification that again take the upper hand. Finally the lung, the lowest of the organs of the upper pole, is, from the fact of its position, the least subject to the upper pole's form-giving forces.

We have noted the affinity of silica with light, which itself plays an important role in tuberculosis. We know that lack of light can favour this disease, and we are aware also of the vulnerability of the tuberculosis bacillus to sunlight and ultra-violet light. We know also the beneficial action of light in properly regulated doses on those suffering from tuberculosis. On the other hand, an excessive exposure to sunlight can be the origin of a particularly severe case of tuberculosis. Rudolf Steiner speaks of a metabolism of light, for light penetrates the organism and undergoes a metamorphosis. Just as our food has to be metamorphosed before absorption into our organism, so must light also be transformed in order to be assimilated. This metamorphosed light also has a bactericidal power. If the organism possesses enough of it, the bacilli are unable to develop. It can happen that a lack of external light is the cause of the lack of metamorphosed light, but more frequently it is the organism itself which is incapable of carrying out this metamorphosis as a result of an inadequate action of the ego in the skin. It is in no way surprising, then, that a person whose skin, the organ of metamorphosis of light, has suffered damage from an immoderate exposure to the sunlight, becomes incapable of properly carrying out this transformation, and so is particularly liable to a massive bacillary invasion. This double aetiology, of either insufficiency of light or an incapacity to metamorphose it, we have already met in studying rickets.

In the treatment of tuberculosis we try especially to strengthen the form-giving processes arising from the upper pole. With this object in view it is not a bad thing for the patient to have to carry out rigorous thought training, for example by working at geometry. We can restrain the tendency of the metabolic pole to overflow by reducing the amount of food. It is a fundamental error to overfeed a tuberculous patient. We act on the process of light metamorphosis by giving *Phosphorus* 5x on waking. Nevertheless phosphorus must be stopped during the months of April, May and June, for it could cause haemoptysis. We can replace it during this period by *Magnesium phosphor* 6x. We stimulate the processes of incarnation by means of iron, which we give in the form of *Ferrum rosatum* 3x, a preparation which associates the petals of red roses with iron. It is a good thing to give *Graphites* 15x at the same time, as this also supplies form-giving forces. We therefore prescribe *Ferrum rosatum* 3x/*Graphites* 15x aa dil. in a dose of ten drops three times a day. We prefer to give patients with a high colour *Ferrum chloratum* comp. *(Ferrum sesquichloratum* 3x/*Graphites* 15x*)*. Equally we make use of the formative forces of silica which may be given with advantage in the vegetable form of *Equisetum*. One must never forget to treat the liver at the same time with *Chelidonium* or Hepatodoron *(Fragaria/Vitis)*, for there will then be less tendency for metabolic products from this organ to overflow towards the lung.

A fourth 'birth' takes place towards the age of twenty-one, the birth of the ego. This age has not been randomly chosen as that for attaining one's majority, for it is only by exercising control of the ego that an individual is able to assume his responsibilities in full consciousness. Thought is still strongly coloured by the emotions between the ages of fourteen and twenty-one, and it is only after the ego becomes free that one has the ability to become really objective, something that cannot be achieved through compulsion!

In the evolution of the individual there are further seven-year developmental periods, but these have a much less direct connection with the art of medicine and we will not enter into them here. We would point out, however, that the gifts which we bring with us at birth will out of themselves allow us to develop only till about twenty-eight years of age. What we become after this age is the result of the work which we are free to do on our own development. It is not surprising, therefore, that some people never exceed this age mentally.

Part Three

THE FOUR CARDINAL ORGANS

For a long while a dominant role has been attributed to certain organs or groups of organs, which have been named cardinal organs. They have been traditionally related to the four natural elements—earth, air, fire and water—and thus with the four different temperaments. Anthroposophy shows that these organs can also be connected with the four constituent elements of man. All these relationships can be summarized in the table below.

CONSTITUENT ELEMENTS	CARDINAL ORGANS	NATURAL ELEMENTS	TEMPERA- MENTS
Ego	Heart	Fire	Choleric
Astral body	Kidney	Air	Sanguine* or nervous
Etheric body	Liver	Water	Lymphatic or phlegmatic
Physical body	Lung	Earth	Melancholic

*The term 'sanguine', used by Rudolf Steiner, can lead to confusion, certain classifications using this word to designate what we refer to as choleric. I shall therefore use the designation 'nervous' as Steiner relates his 'sanguine' temperament to the nervous system.

Knowledge of these connections permits a better under-standing of the pathology of these organs. We shall try to show to what degree observation will allow us to confirm these relationships, and we shall describe for each of these organs several typical diseases in both their physical and mental manifestations.

We have seen in Chapter 4 (pp. 41–2) that a pulmonary affection can show itself on three levels—the etheric or functional, the physical, and the astral or soul level. We shall endeavour, in the course of the descriptions that follow, to connect these different levels and to show in particular how each organ functions as a 'mirror of the soul'. This will enable us to find new therapeutic approaches.

10
THE LUNG

Because of its respiratory function the lung would appear to be an 'air organ', but what is of importance here is not so much the substance that penetrates the organ as the role that it asserts in the organism. For the lung is particularly the organ that puts us in a direct connection with the outside physical world. The digestive apparatus, for example, does not present such immediate relations with the outside world, for the food is transformed when it reaches the interior of the organism, but this is not the case with air. The lung does not start to function until we come into the world, until we become terrestrial beings, and it is therefore also an organ connected with incarnation.

At our first inhalation the astral body unites with the physical etheric complex and at death, at the last exhalation, it leaves the body for ever. At each inhalation this union between the upper and lower complexes is intensified, to be relaxed at each exhalation.

Such considerations make us already inclined to think of the lung as an 'earth organ', but there are others. The lung is strongly connected to the nervous system (and thus to the cold pole of the organism). This can be clearly seen in the development of the embyro and also in the functional regulation of the organ, which is much more closely dependent on the nervous system than is the heart. It is this which allows us to modify our respiratory rhythm at will.

The lung is also a cold organ whose temperature is about 35.5°C; cold is also a characteristic of the element earth.

Finally the lung, by its function of regulating the CO_2 level plays a part in the metabolism of carbonates and especially of calcium carbonate, which is a typically 'earthly' element. The deposition of chalk in the oyster shell, for example, is the polar reflection of an intense living vitality in the oyster. In fact we give *Conchae* (*Calcarea carb.*) itself to those who have a tendency to excessive development of their vital processes— to the detriment, of course, of consciousness.

If the lung is an earth organ, it is nevertheless necessary that the expression of its earthly nature should remain within physiological limits. If the limits are exceeded, conditions such as asthma develop. In asthma we find spasm within the respiratory function. The air is trapped in the pulmonary alveoli, because the astral body is united too intensely with the lung. The patient gives the impression of being *afraid* to breathe out; such anguish is a typical manifestation of the astral body. The retained air impedes inspiration. The over-intense union of the astral body and the lungs gives rise to a 'pressure' on the organ, this in turn giving rise to the secretion of plugs of mucous which further embarrass respiration. Bearing in mind that excretion in the organism is a function of the astral body, secretory gland function, in the proper sense, is an expression of the etheric body. We find that the mucous plugs secreted in attacks of asthma are solid and built up in the shape of Curshmann's spirals or of Charcot-Leyden crystals. These are a result of a process of mineralization, of an excessive '*earth*' tendency, and the spasms then appear as an attempt by the astral body to overcome this hardness or abnormal stiffness. In asthma we observe a process which is normal at the cephalic pole displaced into the lung where it becomes pathological.

Indeed, when we think, we *crystallize* an idea, and we *retain* it and structure it thanks to the activity of the astral body. It is abnormal when such processes work at the level of the lungs, where the exchange with the outer environment ought to take place in a rhythmical and harmonious manner.

These pathological processes that we see in asthma are the reverse of what we have observed in tuberculosis. In tuberculosis a process that should act normally at the metabolic pole has become displaced into the lungs. In tuberculosis we see the destruction of form, tissues are broken down and an abnormal bacterial life appears. By contrast, in asthma spasmodic phenomena occur and processes of mineralization with hardening of structure become manifest. The lung becomes as it were too *earthy*. We can observe the same polarity in the psychological states of those affected by these polar conditions. The tuberculous patient, as mentioned earlier, has a characteristic imaginative life and lack of concern with his condition. The asthmatic, on the other hand, is characterized by his anxiety and by his withdrawal into himself. Characteristically the tuberculous patient seems younger and the asthmatic patient older than he really is. It follows from this that the mineralizing process which produces healing of the tuberculous focus also gives rise to a more rapid ageing than normal of the whole organism.

We often also find an allergic state in the genesis of asthma. Now one can regard this condition as a displacement of metabolic functions into the nerve-sense poles to which the skin belongs. This would seem to contradict what I have already said about asthma. Really, however, we are faced once again with a pendulum-like swing; a process that has developed as far as possible in one direction can produce a swing back in the opposite direction. The further the pendulum swings one way, the greater becomes the tendency for it to swing back the other way. It is therefore not surprising to find asthma occurring when an allergic condition has been 'driven inwards' instead of being healed. The same remark holds good for an onset of asthma after influenza, pneumonia or even tuberculosis, particularly when these conditions have been treated with antibiotics.

There are still some cases of asthma in which the genesis of the disease differs from those we have mentioned above, i.e. cases where the cause is situated at the metabolic pole. Such conditions occur in people of a 'digestive' type, in whom the spasms caused by the astral body are really a reaction to a severe overloading of the organism from the metabolic pole. These patients can be likened to those who suffer from chronic bronchitis, a disease often associated with asthma. Steiner indicated three basic remedies for the treatment of asthma, to be administered by subcutaneous injection:

(1) *Prunus spinosa* 5x to be injected in the neck;
(2) *Nicotiana* 10x to be injected at the costo-vertebral angle;
(3) Gencydo 1–3% to be injected between the shoulders.

These subcutaneous injections are administered in succession in the order given above at two-day intervals, that is, three injections in a week.

Prunus spinosa, sloe or blackthorn, possesses a surplus of vital forces which are not exhausted in the rapid growth of the plant. These forces come to the assistance of the etheric body. This plant is also particularly suitable for patients who are exhausted and drained of vitality.

Nicotiana acts particularly on the *air organism*, which is why this plant is smoked habitually. The leaf of the tobacco plant has an internal zone of a spongy appearance indicating its relationship with the element air, which sustains the astral body. Rudolf Steiner said of the tobacco plant that it corrects the 'deformation of the astral body'. This remedy should be injected at the level of the kidneys which, as we shall see later, are the 'air organs' in which the astral body is especially active.

Gencydo is composed of lemon juice and mucilage of quince and has a selective action on mucous membranes, which it strengthens and makes less irritable. It is also the specific remedy for hay fever, which we shall discuss in detail later.

To complement the injections, Rudolf Steiner recommended giving *Quercus cort.* 10% dil., ten drops in the morning, and *Veronica off.* at night, either as an infusion or as a 10% extract in a dose of ten drops. *Veronica* helps the astral body to free itself and so promotes sleep, while the *Quercus* acts rather in the same way as *Conchae*.

It is sometimes difficult to manage without an antispasmodic in an acute attack, particularly if the patient is accustomed to its use. It can be replaced by an injection of *Lobelia* 6x, the fruit of this plant having the form of a bladder-like capsule which imitates the process of air which we have observed in asthma. Like the tobacco plant, this plant also has a relationship with the air organism and is sometimes smoked by North American Indians. *Belladonna* 3x by injection relieves the spasm, especially in children. In long-standing and very obdurate cases it is as well to start treatment with sulphur baths (potassium sulphate, or *Kalium sulph.*, 30%, one dessertspoonful to the bath).

After the usual treatment in the manner described above, it is generally necessary to treat the patient in a more individual way in order to consolidate the standard treatment. To do this it is useful to know, in addition to the temperament of the patient, the climate or meteorological conditions which generally precipitate an attack. *Blatta orientalis* is given to patients who are sensitive to damp heat, *Conchae* and *Arsenicum album* to those sensitive to cold, and *Apis* to those sensitive to heat, etc. It is not uncommon to see such a treatment of asthma provoke an acute febrile condition, sometimes quite severe. This shows that one is on the right track towards a cure, and more than ever one must be able to respect such a fever. Sometimes an eczema will reappear and this must always be treated with great discretion. I have personally cured a good number of asthmatic patients in this manner, of whom a large proportion were children. It is a great joy for the doctor to see these sickly children, whose heads often appear pushed down between their shoulders, gradually becoming freed from a life of suffering, catching up on their education and taking part in sports again.

Although it is not, properly speaking, a pulmonary condition, we will consider hay fever here because of its relationship with asthma. Like asthma it is an allergic manifestation.

But what is allergy? We shall understand more readily if we compare it with a corresponding psychological condition. We can find it difficult to tolerate certain people. We experience a violent antipathy to them and, if we are inclined to anger, the slightest contact with them is liable to fill us with exasperation. We are as it were oversensitive to these people, and this can express itself in words or even in acts of violence. This enhanced antipathy is a manifestation of our emotional state which attempts to make us repulse the other person with all the strength of our astral body; but this deployment of force is so out of proportion to the factors that have provoked it that an outside observer would find this reaction quite out of place. The same holds good for allergy. The reaction of the mucous membrane in the attacks of streaming of the nose is out of proportion to the few grains of pollen that have provoked it. The accompanying sneezing on the physical plane corresponds to anger and antipathy on the psychological plane. It is not then the pollen grain which should be blamed but the constitution of the person who reacts in such an explosive manner. Violent reactions of the astral body, giving rise to cramps or spasms, are nearly always a sign of weakness, such as we have described by analogy with the alpine climber who clings more strongly to the rock as he feels himself growing tired (p. 54).

The treatment of hay fever, therefore, has the aim of strengthening and harmonizing the action of the astral body in its relation to the mucous membrane. Rudolf Steiner has proposed for this purpose Gencydo (*Mucilago cydonia/ Succus citri*). At the time of its flowering the lemon tree is the seat of an intense process of dispersion, manifest in the form of a somewhat sweetish perfume. This process of dispersion is followed by an opposite process of concentration in the fruit. This centripetal tendency does not go as far as the concentration and dessication we find in grains but gives rise to the formation of a fruit, bringing the etheric forces into play in a distension controlled and limited by the rind, which has an almost leathery texture. These astringent properties are also apparent in the formation of acid rather than sugars. In using the lemon in treatment we show the organism the path that it ought to follow and we give it a pattern. For the mucous membrane ought to be resistant, and neither let the fluids disperse nor allow them to dry up. It should remain 'succulent'. The quince is a rough, hard fruit whose properties reinforce those of the lemon. It has a retarded process of sugar formation, but in this case the result is the production of mucilage whose role in the mucous membranes is already known to us.

Gencydo is administered in the form of subcutaneous injections at the level of the subspinous fossa of the shoulder blade, twice a week. It is important to start these before the appearance of hay fever, i.e. at the end of March or the beginning of April. A second course of ten injections is given in the autumn. Nasal insufflations of Gencydo liquid are given with these injections, most easily with the aid of a nebulizer; but, as this liquid is rather thick, it should be diluted a little. It is important that the whole of the nasal mucous membrane should be moistened with Gencydo. One should see an improvement, often spectacular, in the state of the patient even in the first year. The treatment is pursued for three years. In the first year ampoules of 1% Gencydo are given and in the second and third years ampoules of 2% or even 3%. If the treatment is carried out correctly, it is rare for the condition not to be completely cured by the end of the third year.

We have compared hay fever and asthma because their allergic aetiology and spasmodic nature justifies a somewhat similar treatment, but it should be remembered that from other points of view these are opposite conditions. In hay fever there is an obvious strong centrifugal tendency, but in asthma we have described a centripetal tendency which may go as far as mineralization apparent in crystal formation. The lung, which has a tendency to become too solid, too 'earthy', will be kept from harm by Gencydo, which helps it to preserve its 'succulent' character.

While the function of the lung consists in a constant exchange with the physical world, in the realm of the psyche its role is to give reality to emotional contact with people around us. As we have already seen, social contact is also a form of respiration. A functional disturbance (cf. p. 42) of the organ prevents it from fulfilling its role as 'mirror of the soul' and so hinders normal relations with other people. Such a disturbance can be constitutional and become manifest in the temperament. It may appear only in later life and can then become the cause of psychological conditions.

When the lung, the 'earth-organ', has a certain preponderance over the other organs, the whole organism tends to be dominated by the 'earth' principle. The body then becomes heavier, more physical than it should be, and the ego-astral complex experiences a certain difficulty in incarnating. The superior elements then find themselves in the position of a person who is using a hammer which is too heavy in relation to his strength. This calls forth an effort disproportionate to the object to be attained.

The physical body of the 'lung-man' is truly heavy, dense and slow. His tread is weighty as if he were carrying round balls of clay on his shoes. His head is often bowed and his back bent as if drawn down by the earth. This is the typical physiognomy of the melancholic temperament. To be burdened with a body which he does not succeed in entirely mastering is a source of difficulty and suffering for the melancholic, so that he also has a tendency to retire within himself. He fears his surroundings and is afraid of the crowd. Nevertheless it is not uncommon to see him prefer the anonymity of the large store to the little shop which necessitates a more intimate contact with those serving in it.

When these tendencies become accentuated and assume a pathological character, mental symptoms appear, for example agoraphobia. Such patients crossing an open space may feel deprived of all protection, and this can be a real torture. Introversion becomes more marked and the mind can be filled with daydreams which tend to be systematized rather than varied. Their static character shows itself in thinking in the form of fixed ideas from which the subjects cannot free themselves, although they are conscious of their absurd character. This 'retention' of ideas reminds us of that of air in asthma. Finally they may sink into a profound melancholy or pass into a state of systematized delusions.

In the treatment of mental conditions related to the lung one should first consider hot sulphur baths. *Sulphur* or *Hepar sulph.* can also be given. *Sulphur* activates the metabolism and helps to combat the tendency to hardening. The specific treatment is mercury, the great mobilizer, in the form of *Mercurius per Nasturtium* (0.1% or 1%) + Pulmo by subcutaneous injection over the thorax two or three times a week.

We should also note Rudolf Steiner's[1] recommendation that those of a melancholic temperament should be encouraged to take an interest in the sufferings of others. This helps to prevent them from withdrawing too much into themselves. He also recommended that children with this temperament should be given plenty of sugar in their diet.

11
THE LIVER

Embarking on the study of the liver is rather like penetrating into a tropical forest. The damp humidity characteristic of the rain forest is also characteristic of the liver. An essentially venous organ, the liver is so rich in fluids that it contains little more solid matter than the blood. It is also the heat centre of the body, with a temperature above 40°C. In contrast to the lung which, with its bronchial tree, shows a finely differentiated form, the liver is soft and rather lacking in structure. In contrast to the kidney it possesses a considerable regenerative capacity. Experiments have demonstrated total regeneration after 80% of it has been removed. This capacity reminds us of the vitality of the vegetable kingdom. In both English and German the word which denotes the liver is derived from the verb 'to live'. This shows that in past times people instinctively felt the connection between this organ and life. It is probable that the French word for liver, *foie*, is not derived from *ficatum*, that which is crammed or gorged with figs, but from *ficator*, the root of which we find in the word *végétal*. On the other hand, is not the fig tree the 'tree of life'? As we are speaking of etymology, let us recall that the French word *figer* signifies 'to have the consistency of liver', which brings us to the boundary between the two processes 'solve' and 'coagula' of the alchemists, i.e. between the liquid phase and the solid phase. Many other facts show the role of the liver in the metabolism of water: its action on diuresis, its dysfunction in serous effusions and its role in oedema and the ascites of portal hypertension. This last stems from a deeper disturbance than a mere mechanical difficulty. Finally, a test such as that of induced opsiuria furnishes an experimental proof of these connections between the liver and water. This liquid phase is essential for the manifold chemical activities that are carried on in this organ. The liver is, therefore, the centre of the 'water organism', the medium of our etheric body. It is no way surprising, then, as Rufolf Steiner said and Schwenk[1] has proved, that the liver is strongly influenced by the quality of the water of the region in which we live.

Is the liver chemist or alchemist? Inasmuch as, to a greater degree than any other organ, it is the seat of processes similar to those of nature, and to the extent that, as Steiner has said, it is an enclave of the outside world, the liver is a chemist. That is why it is relatively easy to demonstrate the processes of the liver by current laboratory methods. But the liver is also an alchemist in that the etheric forces take part in these transformations. Glycogenesis and glycogenolysis are examples of this. In glycogenesis the liver transforms the glucose of the blood into glycogen, an insoluble substance closely related to amidon, which it stores up. In glyco- genolysis the glycogen is transformed again into soluble glucose. These processes, which are a typical example of 'coagula' and 'solve', alternate according to a precise rhythm which is independent of mealtimes. Glycogenesis, a process of assimilation, takes place at night or, more exactly, it starts at 3 p.m. and attains its maximum about 3 a.m. The opposite process of glycogenolysis, which is a form of disassimilation, starts about 3 a.m. and attains its maximum about 3 p.m., and is thus diurnal. It is interesting to note that similar pro- cesses are found in the formation of amidon and sugars in plants and this brings us back again to the vegetable king- dom, to the etheric forces and tropical forest evoked above. The fact that the liver possesses, in addition to the arterial and venous circulation which we find in all organs, a portal cir- culation which provides it with a supplement of CO_2, also connects the hepatic processes with those of the vegetable world and especially with those of the leaf.

Let us now turn to the other aspect, that of warmth. Here also etymology gives us an idea of what popular wisdom knew instinctively, without any need of thermocouples! In Russian the liver is called *pyetchen*, which comes from *pyetch*, the stove which is a central element of the Russian house. The metabolism of fats and the biliary processes are connected with this caloric function. The bile contributes, with the pancreatic lipase, to the digestion of fats, substances which are necessary for the maintenance of body temperature. The secretion of bile, a process connected with the breaking down of foodstuffs in the digestive tract, also follows a day and night rhythm, parallel to that of glycogenolysis, starting at 3 a.m. and attaining its maximum about 3 p.m. The bile accumulates in the gall bladder to be utilized according to the requirements of digestion.

The fact that these two functions, regulation of glycogen and secretion of bile, follow a rhythm that is independent of the times of meals confirms our conception of the liver as an enclave of the outer world.

Humidity and heat, these two elements which have served us as a guide in the physiology of the liver, also dominate its pathology. We thus find diseases characterized by an excess or an insufficiency of humidity and by an excess or insufficiency of heat.

If the liver can no longer regulate and control the metabolism of water, then there is a tendency for the water to set itself free, and it becomes like a foreign body for the organism, that is, it stagnates and does not circulate properly. Then we see the appearance of oedema and serous effusions. As these appear more or less distant from the liver, one does not consider this organ as a possible cause of the swelling, but searches for some more or less hypothetical local aetiology.

The proof of the role played by the liver in such effusions is furnished by a therapeutic test. Under certain conditions these effusions can become the seat of reactionary inflammatory processes, for the stagnant fluid acts as a foreign body and the organism tries to get rid of it by inflammation (cf. Chapter 6). We observe the opposite process in cirrhosis, which it would be more correct to call hepatic sclerosis. This condition is characterized by a hardening of the liver, i.e. the 'coagula' takes precedence over the 'solve'. The liver is then unable to carry out its role of vitalizing the fluids and this gives rise to stagnation in the form of ascites. Synovial effusions and arthroses are also disturbances of water metabolism with which the liver is intimately concerned. Such loss of form, whether it arises from excess of fluid or from hardening of the articular and periarticular tissues, is amenable to treatment of the liver.

Disturbances of biliary function are related to the element of heat. Take, for example, catarrhal jaundice. It is not uncommon to find that patients with this condition have overindulged in fats or have used fats of poor quality. When the organism is no longer able to metabolize them correctly, they become 'foreign bodies' and create 'parasitic heat centres' (Rudolf Steiner). These are a source of nourishment for certain viruses, or the centres for the appearance of inflammatory processes. The connection of hepatitis with heat also explains its greater frequency in summer and in hot countries. These inflammations are accompanied by an influx of blood at the liver level, giving rise to an increased production of bile. Owing to a fact which seems paradoxical, this increased production cannot flow away by the biliary passages. What happens is like a fire in a cinema in which the bewildered spectators block the exits. The bile then flows back towards the blood and spreads throughout the whole organism, giving rise to jaundice or icterus.

We see the opposite phenomenon in the formation of gallstones. The liver is then too cold. The production of bile is insufficient and precipitates forms that are deposited in the form of calculi in the biliary passages. The colic which frequently occurs in cases of biliary calculi is the expression of a sudden spasm of the astral body trying to rid itself of the calculi.

Rudolf Steiner inaugurated a new therapy in hepatic diseases, by suggesting three remedies:

Hepatodoron (*Fragaria vesca fol.* 20%/*Vitis vinifera fol.* 20% aa);

Choleodoron (*Chelidonium* 2.5%/*Curcuma rhiz.* 2.5% aa dil.);

Stannum (Tin). He has also thrown light on the action of such plants as *Cichorium intybus* and *Taraxacum*.

Hepatodoron is composed of leaves of the wild strawberry plant and the grapevine. The wild strawberry, which grows in the damp conditions found in open woods (recalling the tropical forest), is characterized by a process of sugar production, which results in the formation of a fleshy receptacle dotted with numerous achenes. In the grapevine we also find a plentiful synthesis of sugars, but this takes place in full light and full sunshine. It results in the formation of the bunch in which each cluster is composed of a number of separate grapes. Nevertheless it is not the fruit but the leaves which are used in the medicine, for in the leaves the processes of development are still fully active. Although these two plants have the active production of sugar in common, they have otherwise polar opposite characteristics, so that Hepatodoron is a remedy which does not act only on one isolated function but on the equilibrium between the different tendencies of the liver. We can prescribe it in all liver conditions and more particularly in those connected with the circulation and the metabolism of water. Symptoms such as thirst and a desire for sugar are pointers towards its use. Hepatodoron is administered three times a day after meals (1–2 tablets).

Choleodoron is composed of *Chelidonium majus*, the greater celandine, and of *Curcuma*. The greater celandine grows near old walls. Its soft, lobed leaves contrast with the hardness of the surroundings in which it is rooted. Its yellow juice recalls bile. The rhizome of *Curcuma* (turmeric), which is one of the ingredients of curry powder, is derived from a tropical plant, and with it we call particularly on the help of the element heat. The character of its components makes Choleodoron the specific remedy for biliary complaints and, above all, for gallstones. It is given by preference after meals in a dose of ten drops in half a glass of warm water or in an infusion. It must be taken for a long period, for at least three years with interruptions of two weeks from time to time, to allow the organism to reassert its own rhythms. The action of Choleodoron is remarkably rapid in the obese type of patient with gallstones, usually fair-haired women who have dramatic attacks of biliary colic. Its action is slower in dark-haired patients of the melancholic type. Having treated more than five hundred cases of gallstones, without having recourse even once to surgical intervention, I consider myself able to affirm both the efficacy of this remedy and also the methods which have permitted its discovery.

The action of *Stannum* is to maintain the equilibrium between 'solve' and 'coagula', between loss of form and excessive rigidity. This metal, associated with Jupiter, is both granular and malleable and acts on the soft parts of the organism, enhancing form (in contrast to lead which acts on the mineral elements and the skeleton). Stannum preserves the body both from softening and from excessive hardening and so prevents deformity. It is prescribed for effusions in association with *Bryonia* (*Bryonia* 6x/*Stannum* 10x aa amp.) by subcutaneous injection in the neighbourhood of the affected region. It is used also in the form of an ointment rubbed into the hepatic region in cases of cirrhosis and ascites (*Stannum* 0.4% ungt.). The action of *Stannum* may be reinforced and orientated by the process of dynamization through the plant which we mentioned previously (p. 44). *Stannum per Cichorium* 0.1% acts especially on acute inflammatory conditions of the liver, *Stannum per Taraxacum* 0.1% on chronic and degenerative processes.

We are far from having exhausted the subject of hepatic pathology with the conditions already described. These few typical conditions must serve us as guidelines and help us to find our way towards appropriate treatment in each particular case. What often makes diagnosis difficult is the sluggish nature of diseases of the liver. Liver pain is almost unknown apart from biliary colic, which is in fact a gall bladder symptom. Also, it is not uncommon to see severe hepatic conditions develop over years without attracting the notice of the patient. It is therefore all the more important to understand the 'psychological' symptomatology of the organ.

The 'liver person' is someone in whom the water organism and the etheric body have a predominant influence, and is characterized by a lymphatic or phlegmatic temperament. He is someone of gentle nature who feels at ease within himself as if he were in a warm bath. He shows that inertia proper to liquids which spontaneously return to their position of equilibrium. He is usually a little stout and gives the impression of elasticity. His walk is slow, regular and without heaviness.

When the liver no longer plays its proper role as the instrument of the soul, these characteristics have the tendency to become accentuated. Good humour becomes changed into weakness of spirit and inertia into depression. The patient is obsessed by the fear of losing his well-being and is afraid of life and the troubles it can bring him. Dysfunction of the liver, the organ of life, gives rise to the fear of life, manifesting for example in the dread of a lack of money or of seeing those near him become the victims of some mishap. All that the future may bring becomes the object of anxiety. These patients also have the tendency to be obstinate and argumentative. The most typical disturbance is indisputably depression. Patients who are affected by it become incapable of carrying out the simplest tasks, for these appear to them as insurmountable obstacles.

Pushed to the extreme, this depression becomes a complete loss of will-power. In Chapter 2 we showed the connection between the will and the metabolism. We shall, therefore, not be surprised to know that the liver is capable of giving rise to such conditions. In one of his lectures Rudolf Steiner connects voluntary energy with the reabsorption of bile in the intestine—an excessive reabsorption inflames us and drives us to action; an insufficient reabsorption makes us indolent. Thus in jaundice, in which the bile is driven back in the liver and reabsorption is practically abolished, there is an unconquerable feeling of tiredness. When reabsorption becomes excessive, desire for action can degenerate into mania. This symptom alternates with that of depression in manic-depressive psychosis.

Although he has a predisposition to these conditions, a person of lymphatic temperament has no monopoly on them. Our diet today often gives rise to a state of chronic hepatic insufficiency and is the cause of depressive manifestations which affect so many patients, whatever their temperament may be.

All such manifestations call for a liver treatment such as we have described above. In the 'hot' condition, which is mania, we use principally *Stannum p. Taraxacum* 0.1%/*Hepar bovis* 4x.

In sluggishness of the liver one should also think of iron, either in the form of *Ferrum per Chelidonium* 0.1% by sub-cutaneous injection over the gall bladder, or in the form of *Ungt. Ferri* 0.4% massaged into the skin over the gall bladder.

12
THE KIDNEYS

Physiologists have studied in detail the excretory function of the kidney. We have precise information on the volume of the circulating blood, on the relation between the oxygen content of the blood in the renal artery and the renal vein, on the energy needed by the process of excretion to counterbalance osmotic pressure and the number of calories involved in the circulation of the blood. If we balance the energy used against the energy supplied to the kidney, a deficiency is noted. Part of the energy has disappeared! From this we can conclude that other processes must take place in the kidney apart from the processes of excretion.

Rudolf Steiner[1] in 1920 was the first to draw attention to a second function of the kidney, no less important than that of excretion, namely, that of transforming food substances absorbed from the digestive system and impregnating them with astral forces, in a manner analogous to that in which the liver impregnates them with etheric forces. Generally speaking, when an organ possesses an external function, it also carries out a complementary internal function. If this internal function for the kidney consists of 'astralizing' substances of dietary origin, that is to say of transforming them into 'sensitive substances', then we must find strong connections between the kidneys, the astral body and the air which is the supporting element of the astral body.

As we saw earlier, the processes of excretion are dependent on the astral body. Moreover, in its high oxygen consumption, in its sensitivity to anoxaemia and its lack of regenerative capacity, the kidney closely resembles the nervous system, which is the instrument of the astral body. This relationship exists even in the embryological stage where the kidney first forms. Excitation of the astral body by fear reacts on the kidney, causing frequency of micturition. One can also make an etymological comparison between 'neuron', the nerve, and 'nephros', the kidney. Lastly, it is interesting to note that an animal that is pre-eminently nervous and is also one of the most intelligent animals, namely, the horse, is also particularly liable to kidney disease and to renal colic. When one sees a horse gallop with its mane flying in the wind, one can really feel the strong connection between this animal and the element of air.

Note also that urine secretion varies with the atmospheric (air) pressure. The frequent occurrence of meteorism in kidney diseases is yet another reason for considering the kidney as an 'air organ'.

This air only shows itself in the kidney in combination with the blood. The kidney is above all an arterial organ and the blood in the renal vein contains little carbon dioxide and retains the bright red colour of arterial blood. This is the opposite of the situation in the liver, which is pre-eminently a venous organ. This combination of oxygen with the blood shows clearly that here the astral body, of which oxygen is really the physical medium, acts in union with the fluid element, that is, through the etheric body, giving rise to anabolic processes (cf. Chapter 4). The excretory function on the other hand involves a more direct action of the astral body, a dynamic action from the nervous pole.

Let us consider the anabolic processes more fully. Although they exist in the vegetable kingdom, proteins or albumens are characteristically animal substances, that is to say substances capable of receiving the impregnation of the astral body so that they may underlie sensation and motility. Foodstuffs which have been deprived of all astrality and of all foreign etheric forces in the course of their passage along the digestive tract and which have reached the 'zero point' in their passage through the intestinal wall are then impregnated with human astrality by the kidney. The secretion of urine is the opposite polarity to this process, representing the rejection of what is no longer utilizable by the astral body (and the ego).

Rudolf Steiner gave the name of 'kidney radiation' to this process of assimilation, which is not localized in the kidney alone, which is only its point of departure, but radiates from the kidney throughout the organism, bringing about various activities which we shall briefly describe. We can thus say that this 'kidney radiation' is an indirect action of the astral body, which induces a process of assimilation, whereas excretion is a direct action of an astral body, via the nerve-sense system. We shall now study what happens when this 'kidney radiation' is either too weak or too strong.

Weak kidney radiation results in an inadequate process of protein elaboration. This can often be observed in persons of leptosomal type. The proteins that have been inadequately 'astralized' are then really in the nature of foreign bodies and as such are eliminated by the kidneys. Frequently the inadequate action of the astral body in such people is not found in the lower pole only, but affects also the upper pole. These are poorly incarnated people in whom the whole upper complex—the astral body and the ego—only reluctantly takes possession of the lower, the physico-etheric complex. The consequence of this is, as we now know, an incomplete breakdown of foodstuffs in the alimentary tract and the passage into the blood of proteins which have kept their animal or plant characteristics and which the kidneys endeavour to eliminate. These two factors—inadequate astralization by the kidneys and incomplete breakdown of food in the alimentary tract—are combined to a greater or lesser degree in the majority of cases of albuminuria. We find this aetiology also in the albuminuria of fatigue, in orthostatic albuminuria, in lipoid nephrosis, etc. Other manifestations such as arterial hypotension, slowing of the respiratory rhythm, intestinal fermentation of glucides with eructations of gas and passage of flatus are also very characteristic of this state.

These symptoms all call for iron, the incarnating metal, which will compel the upper complex to take a firmer hold on the lower. We prescribe this metal in the form of *Ferrum sidereum* 10x/*Pancreas* 6x or 3x aa trit. by mouth or in the form of injections. We should also think of arsenic which it will be sensible to administer in the form of *Levico* 3x (naturally combined with iron).

Disorders of excretion—oliguria, anuria and retention of salt—are, on the other hand, signs of an inadequate action of the astral body from its nerve-sense pole. Such symptoms often accompany acute nephritis where we find lesions of an inflammatory type, which are then an expression of a reaction of the metabolic pole.

In such a case it is necessary to re-establish harmony between these two processes at the level of the kidneys. For this purpose we use the common horsetail (*Equisetum arvense*). This plant is rich in silica and sulphur but has practically no roots or flowers, so that the 'salt' process of the root and the 'sulphur' process of the flower interpenetrate the stem, which is the main part of the whole plant. This plant also possesses an 'aerated' structure which directs us towards the 'air organ', which is the kidney. It serves as a model for the kidney of a harmonizing factor between the metabolic (sulphur) forces and the nerve-sense (salt) forces. *Equisetum* is also used in a general way in kidney conditions of all kinds. We prescribe *Equisetum* in 6x (in long-standing conditions 15x), by mouth or subcutaneous injection. In anuria we apply hot compresses to the kidneys, and also wet-cupping. One should also give injections of *Carbo* 15x/*Pancreas* 6x aa in the epigastric region.

When kidney radiation becomes too strong, the process of protein elaboration becomes hypertrophic and is no longer balanced by the form-giving processes arising from the upper pole. We then find the state of affairs described with regard to hysteria (cf. Chapter 4). But there is a further development; in acting too intensely at the metabolic pole, the astral body becomes incapable of harmoniously influencing the physical body via the etheric body. It then tends to dispense with the mediation of the etheric body and acts directly on the physical. This shows itself in cramps, spasms, arterial hypertension, foul fermentation of proteins, constipation and gaseous distension with meteorism—briefly, all the symptoms of an overactive sympathetic nervous system. People of the pyknic type, with a constitutionally strong astral body, are the most liable to these conditions. Kidney diseases characteristic of this type are therefore especially arterial in nature, such as glomerulo-nephritis.

Since kidney pathology poses the question of salt, it is necessary to study its role in the organism. Generally speaking, plants contain little salt (NaCl) but are rich in potassium. This latter, together with the other alkaline bases, is an indication of etheric activity. Sodium chloride, by contrast, is a substance characteristic of 'animated' beings, that is to say bearers of an astral body. Both man and animals are unable to do without salt, and maintain its bodily level steady to a very high degree, regardless of external conditions or dietary intake. Salt must be associated with the astral body. In its absence the astral body would not be able to act on the etheric body and its medium, the water organism. The consumption of salt opens up the way for the astral forces and so awakens consciousness. If, on the other hand, the etheric body and the water organism take precedence over the astral body, consciousness is blurred. Thus children fed on cow's milk, which is richer in salt than human milk, are usually more wide awake than those who are breast fed (cf. Chapter 1). A craving for salt is usually characteristic of a strong affinity of the 'upper complex' for the 'lower complex'. A reduction in the consumption of salt helps to reduce too intense an action of the astral body. It would therefore be inappropriate to prescribe a salt-free diet when the action of the astral body is inadequate. Nevertheless one must act with much discernment because often several different pathological processes are involved in kidney diseases.

Oedema is often connected with chloride retention. In such a case we may consider it as a reaction of the water organism to get rid of salt in the tissues when the kidneys are no longer able to eliminate it. Not all cases of oedema are of this origin. They are more often an expression of a 'laziness' of the water organism which allows the fluids to stagnate.

So the treatment of an over-strong 'kidney radiation' consists first of all in moderating the action of the astral body and of displacing it from one pole towards the other. We have already called on *Nicotiana* in Chapter 10 to perform this function. *Carbo* is another remedy in this situation. When we carbonize a plant, all that is vital is eliminated and all that is left is the skeleton of the plant, which is carbon. Carbon also has a remarkable affinity with air, not only in its combustibility but also in its property of absorbing gas. *Carbo* is therefore a 'respirator', and helps the astral body to take upon itself the internal respiratory processes of the organism. Meteorism is the principal symptom indicating its use. In kidney conditions we generally use it in a 15x potency. It should also be noted that an injection of *Carbo* 30x will usually bring relief in an attack of asthma of renal origin. By using *Carbo equiseti* we may direct the action of *Carbo* especially towards the kidneys.

Chamomile root is an important remedy suggested by Rudolf Steiner for the treatment of over-strong 'renal radiation'. The root represents the 'salt' pole in the plant and must be related to the nerve-sense system of man, on which it has an elective action. (The flower on the other hand acts especially on the metabolic pole.) The root, moreover, is rich in alkaline salts, directing its action towards the water-organism. From this we can say that chamomile root has form-giving properties in relation to the water organism. We prescribe it whenever there is need to harmonize the action of the astral body on the etheric body. It is a remedy with a wide field of application. We prescribe *Chamomilla radix* in 6x, 15x or 30x potency according to the region in which the symptoms predominate; the low dilutions correspond to the metabolic pole. Let us also recall that *Chamomilla radix* is good for calming mental agitation. We have already seen its use as 4x in insomnia in children.

Excessive nerve-sense activity of the astral body at the level of the kidneys can be the starting point of conditions such as chronic nephritis and nephro-sclerosis. These conditions are often bound up with others and can evolve over years from repeated attacks. The kidney, in contrast to the liver, being incapable of regeneration, the prognosis in these diseases is unfavourable.

In this case treatment aims at strengthening the opposite forces, i.e. those of assimilation. With this aim we use copper. We can employ its oxide, *Cuprite* 4x, or again its vegetabilized form, *Cuprum per Melissam* 0.1%. *Cuprum per Chamomillam* 0.1% is the best choice in cases showing spasms. These two preparations can be given by injection or by mouth. An elegant and effective way of using copper is by application as an ointment at the level of the costo-vertebral angle. *Cuprum*

0.4% ungt. can be prescribed alone or in association with *Nicotiana* as *Cuprum* 0.4% *Nicotiana* 6x aa ungt. Naturally we do not forget *Equisetum* in which we can strengthen the sulphur component by prescribing *Equisetum c. sulfure tostum* in either 4x trit. or 10x dil.

It is customary to separate the pathology of the kidney from that of the suprarenal gland. Yet if we compare the latter with what we have said with regard to the kidneys, we will find many symptoms in common. Hypotension and the asthenia of suprarenal insufficiency remind us of the symptoms of a 'renal radiation' which is too weak. Its excess, on the contrary, can be related to hypertension and the circulatory conditions which are found in overactivity of the suprarenals. All these symptoms are fundamentally the expression of the astral body and call for related therapy.

Although not properly appertaining to renal pathology, it is necessary to say a few words here on the treatment of infections of the urinary tract.

In perinephric inflammations we use Erysidoron 1 and 2 (*Apis* 3x/*Belladonna* 3x and *Carbo* 5%/*Sulphur* 1%) alternately as in inflammation (cf. Chapter 6). We also give injections of *Echinacea* 3x and *Argentum* 20x.

In pyelitis and cystitis, almost always consequent on a chill, one must above all apply compresses soaked in a warm infusion of milfoil or, better still, one gives a hip-bath to which the same infusion has been added. *Cantharis* comp. Wala[2] is a very effective remedy which can be administered either by mouth (ten granules three to six times a day), or by injection in the lower part of the abdominal wall (two or three times a week). This treatment must be carried out for a minimum of ten consecutive days, sporadic or irregular administration causing loss of efficacy. *Cantharis* 4x on its own by injection is an effective first measure in the treatment of cystitis, the injection being given in the lower part of the abdominal wall. One should also think of *Argentum nitricum* 20x.

As the opposite of inflammatory conditions we have renal calculus formation, in which the processes of mineralization arising from the upper pole extend to organs in which they are out of place. The composition of calculi is unimportant, the organism precipitating the substances at its disposition at the time (urates, phosphates, oxalates or carbonates). What is important is the development of an inorganic process of mineralization. It is not uncommon to see this condition in a small child as the result of an untimely administration of vitamin D, which may even be fatal. It is interesting to note that patients with renal calculi often seem to be of the same type, to such an extent that it is sometimes possible to suspect this condition at first sight.

The remedy that Rudolf Steiner suggested for this condition, Renodoron, is composed of flint and the calcareous concretions of the crayfish (*Lapides cancrorum* 15x/*Silica* 15x aa). By its colloidal form flint approaches the organic world and acts on the water organism. *Lapides cancrorum* is a calcareous concretion which appears in the gastric region of the crayfish before it discards its old shell. The crayfish then dissolves these calculi again rapidly to mineralize its new shell, and that is why they can be employed as a remedy in lithiasis. Thanks to Renodoron I have never been obliged to have recourse to surgical intervention in a case of renal calculus.

In the case of an acute attack of renal colic, three cupping glasses should first of all be applied, either in the lumbar region or at the point on the abdomen corresponding to the ureter, depending on where the pain is localized. This simple act will often relieve an attack within a quarter of an hour. One can also use very hot applications. Sometimes it is necessary to give a subcutaneous injection of *Belladonna* 3x/

Oxalis 3x aa. at the site of the pain. These measures usually make recourse to opiates unnecessary. If one is in doubt between the diagnosis of an attack of renal colic or lumbago, one should remember that a patient with lumbago seeks relief in immobility and one suffering from renal colic in movement.

Assimilation and excretion, the two aspects of the renal process, constitute a kind of respiratory rhythm. They resemble a metamorphosis, at a deeper level, of pulmonary inspiration and expiration. We have already drawn a parallel between this latter rhythm and the interplay of sympathy and antipathy (see endnote 3 to Chapter 10). Nevertheless these two sentiments are characterized by some degree of consciousness which we no longer find in the psychological manifestations which we can associate with the kidney. Everything is deeper, more 'organic' at this level, and in consequence less conscious. Thus we associate the kidney with the deep emotional life in so far as it is an instrument of the soul. Thus fear of 'renal type' will be an 'organic fear'. Such people are afraid of having some hidden illness and cancerophobia may also be a symptom of unnoticed renal dysfunction.

Sympathy and antipathy are movements directed towards the exterior. What do they become in their renal metamorphosis, that is to say, when they are directed towards the interior? This dynamic of acceptance or refusal has repercussions in the depths of our being on the state of our soul, which is reflected in our temperament.

The kidney being an 'air organ', we find the mobility of the air element in the temperament of people of the renal type. They are lively but unstable and changeable in their emotions. They follow sudden shifts of the wind like a weathercock, and tend to flit from one thing to another. They are easily pulled in opposite directions, resulting in a tendency to indecision and even, at a deeper level, a schizoid tendency. But mobility also has advantages. On the level of thought it gives rise to vivacity of intelligence. Here we have the opposite of the fixed idea of the melancholic. Nevertheless this intelligence remains cold, passion does not enter into it, and the fire it shows is the flaring of a straw fire or the brief exuberance of a firework.

In his physical appearance the person of nervous or sanguine temperament is rather thin and tall, with a triangular face, the point being directed downwards. At times he gives an impression of buoyancy and his step assumes the nature of a dance. The ease with which he tires makes him quickly collapse into apathy. He may be walking about with his head in the air at one moment and at the next be collapsed in an armchair.

A 'superficial' lesion of the kidney, if it does not allow the kidney to take on its task as instrument of psychological life, can, if it is persistent, become the cause of serious conditions. What in one of a nervous temperament was only a schizoid tendency can become schizophrenia. What was a disturbance of assimilation on the physical plane may become an inability to 'digest' or to assimilate certain events. It is not protein but psychological matters which behave as foreign bodies in the depths of the soul. It is, moreover, not uncommon to find abnormalities of the blood proteins in these patients. The ego no longer occupies the centre of the soul, and everything becomes organized, at first very logically, around these 'mental parasites', which are undigested memories or experiences. We are faced with a condition in which the astral body predominates over the ego, which has become incapable of setting the contents of the psyche in order. These patients are almost always intelligent people, and their reasoning is logical. But it is crystallized round a dominating idea which is not based on reality (and may also vary from time to time). In taking their histories one often finds intellectual precocity associated with premature physical and moral ageing. We shall have occasion to speak of this again in relation to cancer.

To such patients the principal remedy is copper, the metal of assimilation, in the form of *Cuprum per Melissam* 0.1%/ *Renale* 4x aa, by subcutaneous injection at the costovertebral angle. In the case of cramps, spasms and raised blood pressure this is replaced by *Cuprum per Chamomillam* 0.1%/ *Renale* 4x aa. As in all kidney conditions we must think of *Equisetum* and of *Carbo*. One can, for example, prescribe *Carbo* 30x/*Equisetum* 20x aa by subcutaneous injection or again *Carbo equiseti* 20x or 30x. The application of *Cuprum* 0.4%/*Nicotiana* 6x ointment carried out regularly is often very effective. Lastly an attempt is made to give these patients a certain 'weight' by prescribing *Plumbum*, in the form of an ointment (*Plumbum* 0.4% ungt.) which is applied over the splenic region. When one wishes to direct the action of copper towards the nervous system one can make use of its natural silicate, dioptase (*Cuprum silicicum nat.*) in principle in high dilution. One must not forget that these patients are generally lacking in warmth. One must, therefore, ensure that they are adequately clothed and prescribe *Apis* for them, should the occasion arise.

13
THE HEART

The heart is the central organ of the rhythmic system and also of the whole human being. It cannot properly be understood if we consider it in isolation, for it forms a functional whole with the rest of the circulatory system—arteries, veins, capillaries and blood.

We have seen above (Chapter 2, pp. 22–3) that the heart should not be likened to a pump. This false comparison is so fixed in us by teaching received since early childhood that it is difficult for us to realize that it is not the heart which sets the blood in motion but, on the contrary, the blood that sets the heart in motion. Moreover, besides Manteuffel's experiments already mentioned, those carried out with Starling's preparation prove it for us. This involves bypassing the systemic circulation in a heart-lung preparation by the use of a cannula. When the blood is set in motion in this cannula and reaches the heart, the heart begins to beat even after an interruption of several hours, indeed after several days! Here the pre-eminence of the blood is clearly shown.

In its warmth, its mobility, its role in the exchange of substances in the tissues and its faculty for constant regeneration (a red blood corpuscle lives only for a month), the blood belongs to the metabolic pole and is opposed to the nerve-sense system. The heart is the place where these two polarities meet and which it brings into equilibrium and harmonizes. Starling's preparation, mentioned above, allows one to state further that, when one reconnects the bloodstream in the direction of the heart, this organ reacts in a first phase by an increase in the amplitude of the contractions and in a second phase by acceleration of the rhythm. These two reactions result in an increase in the volume per minute. We are not conscious of such variations in output in our own bodies, but we are perfectly able to notice an increase in heart rate. It is therefore important to know that this must be attributed to an increase in the venous return which is, in turn, subject to fluctuation arising from the metabolism.

The flow of venous blood into the heart gives rise to diastole. This centrifugal process of dilation is followed by a nerve-sense reaction of contraction in a centripetal direction, the systole. In diastole the heart gives way to the forces of the metabolic pole, becomes rounded and tends to lose its shape; in systole on the other hand the forces of the nerve-sense pole contract it and restore it to its proper shape. Diastole and systole are thus the expression of two polarities (see diagram below). These two phases normally alternate in time. We can also see this expressed physically in relation to a person's constitution. In the pyknic type, characterized by the predominance of the metabolism, the heart is rounded, while in the leptosomal or tall, thin type where the nerve-sense pole is dominant, the heart is elongated.

If the increase in output and the increase in heart rate are an expression of the stronger action of the metabolic process as, for example, after a meal or in febrile conditions, its

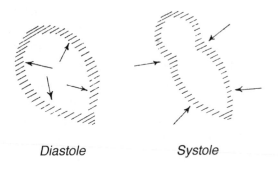

Diastole   Systole

slowing is, conversely, an expression of the more intensive action of the nerve-sense processes. This phenomenon is observed when the vagus nerve is stimulated, as in the oculocardiac reflex when a reduction in heart rate is produced. Similarly, irritation of the meninges, as in encephalitis or in conditions accompanied by a lowering of metabolism, will produce a slowing of the heart. We also note this slowing down in the heart rhythm when severe pain is experienced which is in fact, as we have seen, intensification of the processes of consciousness. On the other hand, when the action of the nerve-sense pole is hindered, the heart rate increases, as we observe in certain forms of bulbar paralysis, in some cases of polyneuritis and in poisoning with substances such as belladonna.

The variations in heart rate during the course of life reflect the same tendencies. In the child, with its very active metabolism, the pulse is rapid, becoming slower with increasing age.

The normal heart rate is 72 per minute, and as the respiratory rate is 18 per minute we may reckon four heart beats to one respiration. This 4:1 ratio tends to be greater in the pyknic and to decrease in the leptosome, possibly to rates of 5:1 and 3.5:1 respectively. These ratios should be looked for carefully when a patient is examined, for changes from normal are a sign of an attempt by the heart to establish an equilibrium between the two poles. It can incidentally demonstrate that the heart is finding difficulty in accomplishing this function. In these changes we have an early and sensitive sign of imbalance which we should be unwise to neglect.

The heart is thus the organ where the two polarities meet, come into opposition with one another and reach an equilibrium. The rhythmic system cannot itself fall ill, as it is essentially harmonious and hence healthy. Certainly the heart, its physical instrument, can be damaged when the compensatory efforts demanded of it exceed its capabilities, especially when these efforts are needed over a long period. Cardiac conditions are therefore the result of the predominance of either the nerve-sense or the metabolic pole. They are thus secondary conditions and often take years to develop, so greatly does the heart strive to re-establish harmony. The observation of established lesions therefore gives relatively little information on the morbid processes involved. It is thus essential to study the development of these conditions over the course of time, which naturally involves taking a detailed case history. Knowledge of these processes will be an incentive for the doctor to try to prevent the development of these cardiac conditions rather than to treat them only after they have developed.

An over-powerful metabolism predisposes to inflammation, but this does not explain why this inflammation is localized in the heart. Such localization is probably never primary, but follows acute articular rheumatism, scarlet fever or diphtheritic or other throat infections. One also quite commonly finds a focus of latent infection, for example in a tooth, which is an expression of a metabolic process not in its proper place and which the formative forces of the upper pole are unable to overcome.

We will now follow such a process in detail and as it were unroll a ball of thread to guide us through the labyrinthine paths of these processes. Let us imagine someone in whom the metabolic pole predominates. Such a person absorbs proteins easily and the upper pole has some difficulty in individualizing them and building them into the organs. When a situation of conflict arises that demands an additional effort at the upper pole, these structuring processes are hindered and proteins of a foreign nature begin to encumber the organism. The body reacts by an inflammatory process, an inflammation of the throat for example, which is an attempt to 'digest' these foreign proteins.[1] If it succeeds in this, all will be well once more; but it can happen that it is only partially successful and then the abnormal proteins persist. These incompletely metamorphosed proteins become deposited in the interstices of the tissues. A heart that is fatigued by such persistent efforts to produce harmony becomes a suitable situation for these proteins to be deposited and thus becomes susceptible to infections, for these incompletely 'humanized' proteins are a favourable medium for bacteria. The heart can thus become a favoured site for infectious processes, and these show themselves by a dissolution or loss of form of the organ. This is what we find in endocarditis, myocarditis and pericarditis. We are familiar with the consequences of these conditions on the anatomical and functional planes.

With these heart infections, or associated with them, one must also consider a morbid process directly connected with the heart's balancing function. When there is present a predominance of the metabolism, the strong current of blood arising from the lower pole has the tendency to over-load the heart, to overfill it. Diastole is to some degree stronger than systole, which arises from the form-giving forces of the upper pole. In the long run the heart yields to this pressure coming from the metabolism and dilates. This process can proceed as far as asystole, if the causes persist. We are presented here, as in infectious diseases, with a loss of form.

The evolution of such a condition is often slow, inter-mittent and insidious. Since a predominance of the meta-bolism over the nerve-sense pole expresses itself by a diminution of consciousness, such conditions are often painless. This explains the frequency of sudden death in these patients who complain so little of their symptoms. It is sometimes necessary to question them carefully to discover slight dyspnoea or over-liability to fatigue, the significance of which must not be overlooked.

Treatment of cardiac conditions due to a predominance of the metabolic pole is essentially prophylactic. In acute articular rheumatism, in scarlet fever, in throat infections and generally in all infections, one must relieve the metabolic pole, that is to say, put the patient on a diet and confine him to bed. These two measures must be continued for several days after the temperature falls during the progress of the illness. It is sometimes difficult to carry them out in children but the doctor must show his authority. Animal protein (meat, eggs) should be avoided also during convalescence, and one should advise against early resumption of the use of salt. The return to a fuller diet should ideally start with stewed apples and rice, which are easy to assimilate.

As muscular activity is a metabolic process, the role of rest in bed is evident. But unnecessary stimulation of the nerve-sense pole must also be avoided, so that it may be in a fit state to carry out its task. Therefore radio, television and even reading should be forbidden. Hospitalization, from the fact that the patient is removed from his usual surroundings and everyday worries, sometimes has a beneficial part to play, but it must be of a good standard and not give rise to additional irritation. Everything depends on the patient's surroundings. In acute conditions isolation is strictly necessary, but in chronic illnesses a shared ward with a good atmosphere can assist recovery. In all illnesses particularly threatening the heart, and especially in cases with a high temperature, Cardiodoron[2] should be prescribed as a preventative.

In infections of the heart we employ *Apis/Belladonna* alternately with *Carbo/Sulphur* (cf. Chapter 6, p. 64). In myocarditis we give *Digitalis* (*Digitalis e fol. digest.* 3x, five drops three times a day); in pericarditis we give *Stannum/ Bryonia* (cf. Chapter 11, p. 125); and in endocarditis lenta we prescribe in the first place a light vegetarian diet containing a large proportion of uncooked items and fruit. We give intravenous injections of *Argentum* 30x and of *Echinacea* 3x (one injection daily of each in turn). We also prescribe subcutaneous injections of *Aurum* 10x/*Stibium* 8x, and *Lachesis* 12–15x.

In all heart conditions of metabolic origin we give as basic treatment Cardiodoron by mouth or by injection and *Aurum* in low potency (10x to 6x). We can also prescribe the metal in the vegetabilized form, *Aurum per Hypericum* 0.1%, this form giving a tonic character to the gold therapy.

At the stage when there is an established lesion or when there is decompensation we give *Crataegus* in addition to the basic treatment and we can prescribe it in combination with the following: *Adonis vernalis* 1%/*Convallaria majalis* 5%/ *Crataegus oxyacantha* 2%/*Scilla maritima* 2% aa. Thanks to the squill, this combination assists in the resolution of oedema. Let us note with regard to *Convallaria*, the lily of the valley, the importance of the rhythmic element in this plant which one could describe as 'musical', for the flowers rise in tiers on the stem like notes on a stave and often form a fifth and sometimes even an octave. We find the same rhythmic appearance in the succession of knots on the root. One is tempted to compare it with Solomon's seal, whose habitat it shares, but in this plant the rhythmic character is more accentuated in the root than it is in the lily of the valley. The forces of heaviness, and thus the element 'earth', are much more marked in Solomon's seal. These characteristics, as well as its more sharply delineated structure, more aerial than that of the lily of the valley, point to the fact that it acts more powerfully on the lung.

In plethoric patients *Carduus mar.* 5% *Paeonia off.* 5% aa (up to 10%, ten drops three times a day) can be usefully employed. The paeony actually rather resembles the chubby face of a plethoric person.

A restricted diet is essential in all cardiac conditions, for the heart is much more often overburdened by food than by muscular work. It is also recommended that treatment should start with an apple cure for one week, followed by three months on a vegetarian diet.

When the heart suffers an excess of the hardening and forming action of the nerve-sense pole, we see effects which are very different from those which result from an excess of the metabolism. Systole then predominates over diastole; the blood vessels, especially the coronary arteries, become sclerosed and narrowed, while arterial spasm reduces the circulation still further. Sometimes a blood clot, which results from an excessive formative process of the blood, completely blocks a blood vessel. Such processes give rise to angina pectoris and to myocardial infarcts from thrombosis of the coronary vessels.

The pain, the anguish and the feeling of impending death are the striking symptoms of these conditions and are in contrast to the painlessness of the conditions of metabolic origin. Generally speaking, precordial pain and cardiac neuroses are the expression of excessive consciousness at the level of the heart. Palpitations, however, are generally the reaction of the heart to a sudden influx of blood arising from the lower pole, and appertain more to conditions of metabolic origin.

It is important to note that angina pectoris and myocardial infarcts affect particularly those who are strongly incarnated, those of the pyknic choleric type. In these cases it is not the constitutional predominance of the nerve-sense pole which underlies these conditions, but the excessive demands made on it by the patient's way of life. Business executives are a typical example. We have a striking confirmation of the influence of the way of life in the following observation of Enos and Holmes.[3] Autopsies were carried out systematically on American soldiers with an average age of twenty-two who fell during the Korean War. They showed 77% of coronary sclerosis, which was apparently related to the intense and repeated stress to which the soldiers were subjected. In contrast, one seldom comes across angina pectoris or cardiac infarction in monks of the contemplative orders, whether they are vegetarians or not.

If in heart conditions of metabolic origin we have given a remedy prepared from a berry, that of hawthorn, in the 'hardening' diseases of the heart we use a remedy originating from a hard seed, that of strophanthus, thereby stimulating in the organism the forces of reaction to this hardness.[4] We prescribe *Ol. Strophanti* 3x, and also give *Aurum*, this time in 30x, possibly in conjunction with *Nicotiania* 10x. In prescribing *Aurum per Primulam* 0.1% we call on a revitalizing aspect of gold therapy. The basic therapy, however, is still Cardiodoron.

In angina pectoris we prescribe *Cactus grandiflorum* 1x–4x and *Magnesium phos.* 3x trit. In cases of infarction we call on the revitalizing property of *Prunus spinosa* 2x–3x in association with *Scorodite* 10x and *Arnica plant tot.* 10x. At the beginning of an attack we give a subcutaneous injection in the left arm of *Arnica plant tot.* 10x + *Nicotiana* 10x, which is usually sufficient to calm down the patient. In thrombosis we would give *Hirudo* 4x combined with arnica. Let us also note the remarkable action of inunctions in the precordial regions with *Aurum* 5x ungt./*Oleum Hyperici* 6% aa, useful both in cardiac neuroses and in more serious conditions.

A true cure of these conditions cannot be obtained without the patient completely transforming his way of life. At first this usually involves absolute rest. This should be followed by a quiet life in which spiritual development gradually takes pride of place over the pursuit of material objectives. An

artistic activity (painting, eurythmy, music, etc.) greatly helps
the patient to recover a harmonious life rhythm.

Human rhythms are related to cosmic rhythms. Some are
under the direct influence of planetary or terrestrial movements. Others, while preserving traces of their origin, have
been interiorized, for example the menstrual cycle, which is a
lunar rhythm but which is no longer dependent on this
heavenly body.

If we consider the respiratory rhythm which is 18 per
minute, we have in 24 hours: $18 \times 60 \times 24 = 25,920$
respirations. This number is that of the duration of the Platonic year expressed in terrestrial years. Let us now work it
out in reverse. If we divide the Platonic year by 12, we get the
Platonic month of 2180 terrestrial years which is the mean
time which the vernal point takes to travel through one
constellation of the zodiac. If we divide the Platonic month by
30, we get 72 terrestrial years, which is the average human life
span. This thus represents a cosmic day. But 72 is also the
average number of heartbeats per minute. In this way we may
understand how the cardiac rhythm is connected with the
solar rhythm.

Only a healthy organ manifests this rhythm. Lesions of
certain regions of the heart make it impossible for it to con-
form with this harmony and are the principal causes of
arrhythmia which may be temporary but is often permanent.
This condition must always arouse suspicion of the existence
of an unrecognized past lesion which should be looked for.

Apart from arrhythmia proper, we recognize disturbances
of rhythm which we have already considered in relation to the
predominance of one of the poles, namely, bradycardia and
tachycardia. We shall consider briefly three forms of tachycardia of which it is interesting to know the causes.

Paroxysmal tachycardia is characterized by attacks of
rapid heart beat. Because these attacks begin and end

abruptly, this condition has been connected with the nervous system. This is not inaccurate if we consider the nervous system as the instrument of the astral body. We are then led to recognize a sudden and momentary suspension of the action of the nervous system, which involves a 'disconnection' of the astral body at a given place in the nervous system, for example a kind of sudden paralysis of the vagus nerve. This instability of the astral body allows very minor causes to start off an attack.

We have the opposite process in emotional tachycardia. In the preceding chapter we showed the relation between emotion and the kidneys. Notice how an emotion is accompanied by a real feeling that something from much deeper down is rising up within one. Does one not say that one feels anger *rising*? There is in fact an afflux of blood towards the heart in emotional tachycardia. However, owing to the inertia of the blood mass, we do not have the suddenness as in paroxysmal tachycardia. Both the onset of the condition and its resolution are more gradual.

Thyrotoxicosis, Graves' disease, is quite closely related to emotional tachycardia. This condition appears especially as a sequel to an emotional upset. It is the expression of a considerable intensification of the action of the astral body throughout the *whole* organism. That is why some symptoms of this illness show intensification of the action of the astral body at the lower pole (tachycardia), while others show its intensification at the upper pole (loss of weight). This explains the variation in the clinical forms of this disease and certain of its apparently contradictory aspects. The symptomatology of both hypo- and hyperthyroidism gives us a sense of the strong connection between the thyroid and the astral body.

We use copper to moderate and harmonize this influence of the astral body, as *Cuprite* 4x in blondes and *Cuprum sulph. nat.* 4x in brunettes. We say blondes and brunettes because it is nearly always women who are affected. We also give *Nicotiana* 10x and, if there are cardiac symptoms, *Ol. Strophanti* 3x.

We have seen in previous chapters that the liver is the hot pole and the lung the cold pole of the organism. The heart occupies a median position between the two in accordance with its function of equilibration. None of the heat processes of our body is conceivable without the blood and circulation. The heart is also the centre of our 'heat organism', without which the ego would be unable to manifest itself. The blood is thus the instrument of the ego, just as the nervous system is the instrument of the astral body.

In so far as it is the result of combustion, and is thus in reality a process of degradation leaving a mineral residue, ash, heat formation is dependent on the direct action of the ego at the upper pole (cf. p. 25). That is why stimulation of certain areas of the brain can cause fever. But the heat itself appears at the lower pole and then allows the ego, after having associated itself with the astral and etheric forces, to unite with the blood and extend its action throughout the organism from the lower pole upwards. In this way it counterbalances the influence of the nervous system. It is not only physical warmth that we find engendered here but also spiritual warmth, the warmth of enthusiasm, of courage, of self-sacrifice, and that of love. It is therefore entirely justifiable to associate the heart with the element fire.

All these forms of warmth are characteristic of the 'heart person', in whom the dominant constituent element is the ego. We are confronted by a strong personality, capable of obstinately pursuing an aim, with a tendency to impose his will by every means, but also inclined to acts of generosity. All depends on the aim to which his will is directed. Applied to thinking, this will enables him to attain the greatest heights. On the other hand this power of will does not easily tolerate obstacles and thus predisposes to anger. A person with such a temperament is physically rather thickset. This is the pyknic type, which lacks the softness and elasticity of the lymphatic type. His gait gives the impression that he wants to stamp his footprints on the earth. His eyes, often very dark in colour, shine with a dull lustre and are quite different from the soft, velvet brown eyes common in people of lymphatic type. His musculature is usually well developed. Napoleon Bonaparte is cited as an example of the choleric type by Rudolf Steiner who adds, however, that he later developed the lymphatic temperament to some degree. Beethoven was certainly a choleric type also.

The supremacy of the ego can change into a need for self-assertion towards and against everything, into the wish to persist in one direction even when it has been recognized as false. What was courage, that is to say action which consciously overcomes danger, becomes sheer rashness. What was will becomes acute mania.[5] This lack of control and liability to wild outbursts is the danger to which the choleric is exposed. It sometimes leads to self-destruction and frequently involves others in its downfall. It is a conflagration which lays everything waste.

When the heart is too strongly influenced by the forces of the nerve-sense pole, there appear cardiac neuroses which are so common in medical practice. An unconscious perception of the catabolic processes arising from this pole show themselves in anguish and fear of death, even where there are no serious lesions that put the life of the patient in danger. It is precisely the 'superficial' conditions of the heart (cf. pp. 41–2 and 108) which are accompanied by such symptoms.

In neurotic manifestations which show an excessive influence from the upper pole we chiefly prescribe *Aurum per Primulam* 0.1 by injections and inunctions in the precordial region with *Aurum* 5x ungt./*Ol. Hyperici* 10%. We also think of *Prunus spinosa* 3x, which has a vitalizing action on the whole patient.

In acute mania, on the other hand, which is an expression of an unleashing of the will forces in relation to metabolism, we employ *Aurum per Hypericum* 0.1%, and possibly *Belladonna* 3x. When faced with a patient in a violent condition we can resort to an injection of apomorphine (five or six milligrams). Inducing vomiting diverts the action of the astral body and with it that of the ego towards the stomach, and the pole of the will is thus curbed. When there are suicidal threats, especially when they are the expression of a tendency to self-assertion that goes as far as self-destruction, *Aurum* 6x–10x is prescribed (or possibly *Aurum per Hypericum*). Cardiodoron is also given in addition to all these remedies.

SUMMARY OF TREATMENT OF CARDIAC CONDITIONS

1. *Predominance of metabolism/will pole:*
   Basic treatment:
   Cardiodoron A
   Aurum praep. 6x–10x
   Aurum per Hypericum 0.1%

   Inflammatory conditions: patient immediately begins a light or special diet.

   Endocarditis:
   Apis 3x/*Belladonna* 3x alternating with *Carbo* 5%/*Sulphur* 1%
   Argentum praep. 30x (inj.)
   Echinacea 3x (inj.)
   Lachesis 12x (inj.)

   Myocarditis:
   As endocarditis + *Digitalis e fol. digestio* 3x (ten drops three times a day)

Pericarditis:
As endocarditis + *Stannum* 10x/*Bryonia* 6x (inj.)

Endocarditis lenta:
Vegetarian diet
Argentum 40x alternating with *Echinacea* 3x by daily
intravenous injection.
Lachesis 12x–18x (inj.)
Aurum 10x/*Stibium* 8x 3:2 (inj.)
Carbo betulae c. methano 3x (trit.)

Valvular conditions, incompetence, decompensation:
Adonis 1%
Convallaria 5%   }   aa dil. ten to fifteen drops three
Crataegus 2%   }   times a day.
Scilla mar. 2%
Carduus mar. 5% *Paeonia off.* 5% aa dil. ten drops three
times a day. Possibly five drops of 10% instead of 5%.

Acute mania:
Apomorphine five to ten milligrams (inj.)
Belladonna 3x (inj.)

Arrhythmias:
Aurum 10x–15x
Cactus 4x
Camphora 3x   }   aa dil. ten drops three times a day.
Sarothamus 1x–2x

2. *Predominance of the nerve-sense pole:*
   Basic treatment:

   Cardiodoron B
   Aurum praep. 30x
   Aurum per Primulam 0.1%
   Ol. Strophanti 3x
   Aurum 5x ungt./*Ol. Hyperici* 10% aa

Angina pectoris:
Cactus 1x–3x
Magnesium phos. 3x (trit.)
Arnica 10x + *Nicotiana* 10x (inj.)

Myocardial infarct:
Arnica e pl. tot. 10x (inj.)
Scorodite 10x (trit.)
Prunus spinosa 3x–6x
Nicotiana 10x (inj.)

Coronary thrombosis:
Hirudo 4x
Arnica e pl. tot. 10x

Cardiac neuroses:
Aurum per Primulam 0.1%
Prunus spinosa 3x
Aurum 5x ungt./*Ol. Hyperici* 10% aa

Exophthalmic goitre (Graves' disease):
Cuprite 4x (blondes)
Cuprum sulphur nat. 4x (brunettes)
Nicotiana 10x (inj.)
Ol. Strophanti 3x

We have attempted to show clearly the characteristics of the four temperaments through consideration of the cardinal organs, the human being's constituent elements and the natural elements. Such an outline is necessarily very schematic and can be but one method of approach. If we want to understand a human being well we must, after having classed him provisionally in one of the four categories, search for everything that characterizes him, that makes him an individual like no one else, a task which no mere computer can accomplish. One must study the person's whole life and his psychological make-up, if one wishes to produce a fundamental cure.

Many of our contemporaries live in fear—fear of the environment in relation to the lung in the melancholic type, fear of life in relation to the liver in the lymphatic type, 'organic' fear in relation to the kidney in the nervous type, and fear of death in relation to the heart in the choleric. One must learn to recognize, little by little, the symptoms of these different fears and to realize their importance, for they are a valuable help in tracing the sources of illness.

Comparison of the four cardinal organs with each other reveals to what extent their functions are interconnected and have repercussions on each other. It is necessary for the sake of clarity to study them separately, but it is only in seeking the dynamic interplay of polarities that it will be possible to understand the whole.

Part Four

SOME SPECIAL PROBLEMS

Considered apart from its underlying concepts, anthroposophical medicine would consist only of a mass of rigid prescriptions applied to rigorously indexed conditions. It is, however, a medicine for the human being and therefore a medicine of the individual. The particular problems to which we shall address ourselves in the fourth part of this book are given only as examples showing possible therapeutic paths, for the first aim of medicine is to cure.

14

THE PROBLEM OF CANCER

If we define cancer as a process of pathological growth, it follows that we shall not be able to understand it as long as we are unable to understand the regulation of normal growth. The difficulties in understanding normal growth can be summarized in two questions: What is growth? And why does it cease? In tackling the pathological aspect it is necessary to pose a third question: Why does growth begin again at a given moment? Finally we also have to ask why it takes on a malignant character and what the reasons are for the localization of a tumour at any particular site.

The first question was posed by the research worker Sir William Savory and the three following questions by Holtzapfel in a masterly study published in 1967.[1] In fact Rudolf Steiner gave us the answers to these questions long before 1967, and excellent studies by Leroi,[2] based on long practical experience, have approached the kernel of the problem. I shall attempt to make a synthesis of these different studies in the light of what we have learned from the early chapters of this book.

We have already given an answer in the first four chapters to the first question—What is normal growth? We have seen that it is the result of two activities, one of multiplicative cell division arising from the etheric forces, and the other of form-building, the sculpturing activity of the forces of the astral body and the ego which transform the etheric forces into *formative forces*. If the forces of multiplication, of reproduction, were to act on their own, the organism would become a vast *morula* (see Fig. 2, p. 12), but a sculpturing force appears at the next stage of embryonic development, the *blastula* stage. It is as if an invisible envelope resisted the centrifugal forces of the morula, holding these forces back. One has the impression that the cells, with their tendency to dispersion, are as it were pressed against this invisible envelope and arrange themselves in a single layer, so forming the *blastula*. There is obviously no envelope in the physical sense of the word. It is in reality the first expression of the sculpturing forces acting in a *centripetal* direction. These forces still act from outside at this stage, and in the plant continue to do so for its whole lifetime. We see, in contrast, these forces interiorize themselves at the *gastrula* stage in animals and man.

Arndt's experiment, as described by Leroi, is a particularly striking example of the action of these two forces, because one sees reproduction and form production follow each other. This is what he says:

Professor Arndt has for a long time observed a little fungus which grows in the woods, called *Dictostelium muconoides*. It is only a few millimetres in height, and is capped by a capsule containing spores. Professor Arndt cultivated these fungi on some broth culture medium. When the fungi are mature, the capsule bursts and the spores fall on the culture medium. The spores develop and amoebae grow out of them. If the culture medium contains bacteria, the amoebae start to ingest them. After having ingested about ten thousand bacteria, the amoeba starts to divide. The amoeba, being a living organism composed of only one cell, behaves like other cells when they multiply. This process of multiplication continues until there are thousands of these mobile cells. When the food supply starts to fail, an astonishing thing happens—Arndt describes how waves begin to spread in the whole cell culture, and how the cells begin to make for certain points of concentration, where they gradually build up the fungus out of their own bodies. First they form the stem and then the rudiment foretelling the capsule and the spores. Little by little the fungus is seen to come into being, the body being formed by the amoebae themselves. A section shows how the amoebae are transformed into fungus cells, undergoing differentiation according to whether they form the capsule or the stem! ... Professor Arndt was asked what directed the amoebae so that they formed a fungus. He replied, 'The *god* of the amoebae.' This is inaccurate. If one wishes to talk of a *god*, one must say, 'It is the *god* of the fungi.'

It is particularly interesting to see a slow-motion film of this remarkable phenomenon, which makes visible the etheric forces in a most striking way.

We see in the first phase of this experiment that the forces of multiplication, acting in a centrifugal direction, cause the amoebae to proliferate and disperse, while in the second phase the centripetal formative forces—the 'god' of the fungi— direct the amoebae towards a centre and there form the fungus with the aid of the cellular material of the amoebae.

When we isolate cells in order to cultivate them apart from the organism in which they have originated, as in Carrel's tissue culture experiment,[3] we observe exactly the opposite phenomenon—form and differentiation are lost and proliferation is speeded up.

We can therefore define normal growth as a process of multiplication *controlled* by sculpturing forces.

The equilibrium between these two forces is modified during the course of existence. Little by little, structure becomes more definite and more mineralized and takes on a *relatively* greater importance. Thus the organism hardens as it becomes older.

We could imagine that this equilibrium is modified by an increase in the power of the sculpturing forces. In fact nothing of the kind occurs. It is the forces of multiplication which diminish or, more precisely, metamorphose. They are thus able, as we have seen in Chapter 8, to be transformed into thought forces; but they can also be used to transform the function of the organism to whose construction they have contributed. This is what we observe in the testicles and ovaries at the time of puberty. These forces later become free again in women at the menopause when the functions of the ovaries slow down or cease. They must then undergo a new metamorphosis on the spiritual level, and transform themselves into wisdom and kindness.

Parallel with this metamorphosis of the forces of multiplication, we see the redundant sculpturing forces metamorphose so as to underpin thinking; for thinking in its turn has to be structured (see graph, p. 76).

Our answer to the second question is therefore that growth ceases because the forces of reproduction and equally of form production are metamorphosed and made use of at another level.

The third question of why, as we see in cancer, growth can reappear at a given moment relates to pathology.

From what has been said above, we have ascertained that growth can only resume if a disequilibrium arises between the forces of multiplication and form production to the advantage of the former. That is in fact what occurs—there is inadequate metamorphosis of the forces of multiplication and a withdrawal of the sculpturing or form-endowing forces.

This inadequate metamorphosis of the vegetative forces explains a multitude of facts. Thus we can understand the appearance of sarcomas at the time when bone growth finishes. This cessation of growth occurs earlier in girls than in boys as does the formation of bone sarcoma. Tumours of the testicles develop when they are ectopic and cannot become functional, so that the growth forces remain unutilized. Cancer of the uterus, breast and prostate arise when these organs cease to be functional and when the metamorphosis of the forces that were used for their function is not accomplished. Thus cancer of the breast is more common in women who have not breast-fed children (cf. pp. 75–6).

Nevertheless the failure of metamorphosis does not necessarily lead to cellular proliferation. It only creates conditions favourable for it. In his first course of lectures to doctors, Rudolf Steiner[4] said that absence or incompleteness of metamorphosis created what he called 'islets of organization' which remained dormant, awaiting favourable conditions. Here we have a conception that is not dissimilar to Cohnheim's theory of dormant 'embryonic islets',[5] but with the difference that this latter theory presupposed the presence of physical residues, while in Steiner's conception it is *forces* (etheric) which constitute the 'islets of organization'.

If thought forces are activated too early in life when the ego is not mature enough to direct the metamorphosis, the etheric forces which are made use of preserve a vegetative character which can manifest itself much later in a propensity to schizophrenia. This premature utilization of the etheric forces explains the lower frequency of cancer in certain mental illnesses.

The etheric residues, which compose these 'islets of organization', will not be stirred into action as long as they are held in balance by adequate form-maintaining forces. If this does not happen, then they realize their potential and produce cellular proliferation.

Inasmuch as they are integrated into the etheric body and have become *formative forces*, these structural forces undergo metamorphosis just as those of multiplication do. But this constitutes only a partial answer to the third question.

In order to understand more fully the interconnection of these facts it is necessary to consider again the direct action of the ego and the astral body at the nerve-sense pole, which shows itself in processes of devitalization, form production and mineralization. If the etheric body, aided by the ego, does not produce regeneration of what has been broken down, foreign material accumulates which the organism tries to get rid of through inflammation. If the disorder persists, the organism becomes gradually resigned to it and the inflammatory processes gradually die down until ultimately sclerosis ensues. But it can also happen that these formative processes arising from the upper pole become still more intense. One could then expect them to cause a 'super-sclerosis'. But nothing of the kind occurs, for life is essentially rhythmic, nothing goes on increasing indefinitely, and when a process exceeds a certain intensity, it undergoes metamorphosis. Here we find the law of the pendulum again. What was a formative force acting in a centripetal direction is transformed, beyond a certain point, into its opposite and becomes a force of dispersion acting in a centrifugal direction. The ego and the astral body then withdraw from the organs, making way for external terrestrial influences.

There is thus a polarity between inflammation and cancer, confirmed by the spontaneous cures that have been observed in the course of acute febrile conditions such as erysipelas. There is a polarity of a different type between cancer and sclerosis. This is confirmed in practice by the fact that signs of sclerosis are rarer in cancer patients than in normal people. Thus sclerosis and cancer are variations of a similar process whereby what normally belongs to the nerve-sense system is extended to the whole organism.

In describing a cancer as an ectopic sense organ, Rudolf Steiner gives a picture which allows what has been said above to be more easily understood. In sense organs, and in a general way in the nerve-sense system, the creation of form is pushed to an extreme at the expense of the powers of regeneration. But something else occurs—it is necessary for the astral body and the ego to withdraw from a sense organ for it to be suitable for perception. A sense organ greatly resembles a physical instrument. The ego and the astral body could no more make use of a sense organ without withdrawing from it than we could use a telescope by placing ourselves inside it.

This is normal at the nerve-sense pole but becomes illness at the opposite pole. By withdrawing from a metabolic organ, the astral body and the ego leave the field free for the unmetamorphosed etheric forces which constitute these dormant 'islets of organization', as well as for external environmental influences.

Our answer to the third question is therefore that proliferation becomes active again when a disequilibrium appears between the sculpturing or form-producing forces and those of multiplication, to the advantage of the latter.

We can now understand why the nervous system, which is highly structured and differentiated, only rarely gives rise to tumours (2% of all cases of cancer) and that these are often relatively benign. On the other hand the premature withdrawal of the form-giving forces from the nervous system is the reason for the relative frequency of these tumours in early childhood. In contrast, cancer is common at the metabolic pole where the processes of regeneration remain very strong throughout life (75% of all cases of cancer occur in the digestive and reproductive organs) and these are often highly malignant.

What is it that makes a tumour malignant? H. Siegmund said that cancer was a 'catastrophe of form'. A natural catastrophe leaves chaos in its wake, that is to say, an extreme degree of disorganization. This is the real situation in cancer. When a metabolic organ becomes an 'ectopic sense organ', that is to say, when the organizing forces of the ego and the astral body withdraw to a greater or a lesser extent, the organ is exposed to external influences and becomes the plaything of chaotic forces. Instead of order maintained by the higher constitutional elements, one sees the inner disorder which occurs so frequently in our modern world. The cells, instead of working together in an orderly way, begin to live a life of their own, to proliferate freely and to fall prey to influences arising from the physical world.

It must be added that these external influences are extremely varied. They can have their source in substances produced in human industrial processes, against which the organism cannot defend itself. By reason of his common origins with the natural world, man is capable of reacting to natural substances. The situation is not the same with synthetic substances, so that against these he is relatively defenceless. For example, natural petroleum is not carcinogenic, whereas the products of its distillation or degradation are so in varying degrees.

Among these external influences must also be included all that penetrates into man through his sense organs (particularly those of hearing) and which slip into the subconscious without having been filtered through conscious perception. Try and recall all the auditory perceptions of a day in a modern city—the noise of cars, aeroplanes, different machines, radio and television sets, etc. You will then realize that only an extremely small part of your perceptions have been the object of conscious apprehension. These forms of attack on your senses, from the modern world, promote the state of chaos which we observe in cancer.

Psychological shocks, well-known as a trigger of cancer, are also a kind of attack on the organism. Leroi cites a particularly striking example of a woman who was suffering from advanced cancer of the bladder.

The tumour at first regressed under treatment. Then the husband of the woman fell ill and had to have a leg amputated. The woman immediately had a relapse of her cancer, and only energetic treatment succeeded in again bringing about an improvement in her condition. The following year the husband died and the woman then had another relapse for which further treatment was necessary and was fortunately effective.[6]

Statistics published in recent years in the USA and in Sweden have shown that cancer is much more frequent in women who have been divorced than in married women. One presumes that this results from the extreme psychological stress suffered in divorce.

Therefore our answer to the fourth question is: malignancy is the expression of a disorganizing action of diverse external influences which the internal forces of organization are no longer able to control.

Cancer is often considered to be a virus infection. It is true that it is possible to cause tumours in animals with the help of oncogenic viruses. But it must not be forgotten that their inoculation is a laboratory procedure which has nothing in common with the situation we meet in life. Nevertheless viruses have been found in cancer cells, but this is not at all surprising when one knows that most viruses—some of which may even be crystallized—are essentially a form of transitional life between the vegetable kingdom and the animal kingdom. One can therefore understand their affinity for tissues whose 'organizing' forces have withdrawn. We can count them among the external influences disposing to cancer. They are not the cause of cancer but increase the disposition to it through their disorganizing influence.

The appearance of the tumour is not the beginning of cancer but a sign of the last phase in its development. When we question cancer patients, we learn that they have often suffered from symptoms for years before the tumour appeared. The tumour itself is really only a sign that the cancer illness has become localized.

The 'islets of organization' mentioned above are one of the causes of localization, but there are many others. Irritation of the skin which, from its repetition or persistence, is no longer accompanied by inflammatory reactions, is the sign of exclusion from the area concerned of the astral body and the ego, thereby creating the possibility of malignant changes. These can even appear in the absence of all predisposition, and are all the more obvious when the form-giving forces of the organism are impaired.

The irritating agent can be mechanical, chemical or even physical, such as burns and ionizing radiations. We know the sites where cancer arises due to tobacco and alcohol. The great frequency of cancer of the stomach in the Japanese is probably not unrelated to their habit of drinking boiling hot tea.

Thanks to the experiments of Druckrey[7] on rats, we know that the yellow colouring matter in butter is capable of giving rise to cancer of the liver. Thus certain substances have a selective action on certain organs. It is interesting to note that in these experiments the liver tumour did not appear until the rats had absorbed a certain quantity of the carcinogenic substance which was constant, and this was independent of the length of intervals during which the administration had been interrupted. From this one can see that the liver truly has a function as a 'sense organ' which 'measures' the dose received. We note also, a point of interest for the prevention of cancer, that the dose of yellow colouring matter in butter needed to produce liver tumour is much higher in rats whose diet included millet. Millet thus has anti-cancer properties, probably due to its content of silica, the element which strengthens the formative forces.

This idea of summation of carcinogenic effect, which we get from Druckrey's experiments, must actively concern us. The food which we eat contains a multitude of chemical products, of which none by itself seems to be absorbed in sufficient quantity to cause cancer—and they are therefore declared innocuous—but it seems almost certain that their sum total goes beyond the safe dose. Here is an example. One knows that benzopyrine is a carcinogen beyond a certain threshold. J. Bornfelt[8] proved that, in the presence of detergents, it is possible to cause cancer of the stomach with benzopyrine in a much lower dose than would be necessary in their absence.

It is often noted that cancer attacks a weak point in the organism, for example an organ that has undergone a surgical operation more or less recently, or the site of some previous trauma. The idea that a blow on the breast can be a factor giving rise to cancer is a classical example.

Without claiming to have exhausted the subject, we have dealt with the principal causes of localization which are: the persistence of islets of organization, trauma (mechanical, physical, chemical and psychological), and in a general way the idea of a point of weakness.

Having answered the five questions that we posed, it remains to study the evolution of cancer in time, and therapeutic possibilities.

Cancer evolves in three stages: a pre-tumour period, a period of tumour growth and a period of metastases. The relative duration of these three periods is extremely variable.

During the pre-tumour period the sculpturing or formative forces are still strong enough to control the vegetative processes. Physical examination is therefore negative, but close questioning and careful observation often disclose a number of facts which become significant only by their association with each other.

Fatigue is one of the first symptoms patients complain of, a rather particular kind of fatigue, different from that which we feel when we have carried out some physical work or even intense intellectual activity, or after a mountain walk. The fatigue of the cancer patient is rather more a lack of animation or initiative. For example, a person who liked reading now closes his book again after the first few pages; or an odd job man begins to let his tools go rusty. These people do not consider themselves ill, they rarely complain, and it is often only those around them who notice a change in their behaviour and urge them to consult a doctor. This kind of lassitude is often noticeable in their expressions. Their eyes appear slightly veiled and their gaze seems to be turned inwards as though they are 'listening internally'.

The medical history frequently reveals the presence of an 'undigested' painful happening as the starting point of these troubles. It might be the loss of someone dear which has never been fully accepted. It could also be the impossibility in which the patient found himself at one point in his life of fulfilling something on which he had set his heart—a young man, for example, who was musically gifted, but had much against his will to give up the pursuit of a musical career to be sure of earning a livelihood.

A symptom not to be neglected is insomnia. One could even say that any insomnia beginning without evident cause must make one suspect latent cancer. As it is common that the patients do not complain of this of their own accord, it is necessary to question them systematically about their sleep.

The lack of previous illness in these patients is striking. They often declare that they have never been ill. This is partly due to the fact that they have suffered but little from febrile conditions owing to their low susceptibility to inflammatory conditions. But their mental make-up also has its part to play, for these patients tend to become less and less communicative. Let us note on this subject that people who suffer from cancerophobia as well as those who are always talking about their own troubles rarely suffer from cancer.

Slowing down of the metabolism is often the cause of *digestive troubles* which need to be investigated—loss of appetite, various manifestations of hepatic insufficiency, atonic constipation, etc. It is not uncommon to note in such patients the beginning of some degree of aversion to meat.

On examination we often note that the skin has a dull look. It is not dry but it gives the impression of 'breathing' badly. The patient sometimes shows scattered spots on the skin, usually naevi which have been present for some time. One also notices particularly the absence of signs of sclerosis, even in patients of a relatively advanced age.

It is extremely important for the doctor to be able to recognize this first phase of cancer, for it is at this stage that treatment gives the best results. The laboratory can furnish very valuable assistance. Recourse is made principally to two methods whose principle was suggested by Rudolf Steiner, that of sensitive crystallization and of the capillary-dynamic picture. We have already mentioned the former which was developed by Pfeiffer and Bessenich (cf. p. 9). The second has been the object of extensive work by Kolisko and has been studied in its application to cancer by Kaelin[9] for more than forty years. It demonstrates particularly well the three stages of cancer, and gives useful indications from the point of view of prognosis. These methods of visualization of the etheric forces reveal a qualitative aspect of the processes. For this reason they give much more valuable information than quantitative methods. They are at present in use throughout the whole world as much for the diagnosis of cancer as for various different qualitative investigations. For the supervision of treatment, on the other hand, the serum copper and iron levels are valuable indicators. In a healthy person their levels vary between 80 and 150. In cancer patients the level of copper rises while that of iron falls. Dr Helmuth Muller of Unterhausen[10] has for some years been carrying out systematic research into these levels in patients treated with Iscador and has shown their progressive return to normal in all cases on the way to clinical improvement. The persistence of abnormal levels, on the other hand, has always been a sign of incipient relapse or metastasis.

We shall not dwell on the second and third phases of cancer as these have been thoroughly studied in manuals of pathology. It is nevertheless necessary to justify this division of its evolution into three stages.

We have seen that in the first stage the vegetative forces were still controlled by the formative or structural forces. In the second period, that of the tumour, the barrier breaks down at a given point in the organism, giving free rein to proliferation. The organism has not, however, abandoned the struggle. One can note, apart from any treatment, a rise in temperature in the area around the tumour, this already constituting an attempt at defence. In the first period, on the other hand, the patient often complains of a sensation of cold in the area in which the tumour ultimately appears. To return to the tumour phase, we recall that many cancer cells have been found in the blood without giving rise to the slightest evidence of metastases. These circulating cancer cells must, therefore, be destroyed by the organism. And another proof of defence by the organism against cancer is that at autopsy, in some patients who have not died of cancer, there have been found groups of malignant cells in the prostate or in the thyroid, and this in the absence of all clinical symptoms of cancer. These groups of cells have therefore been held at bay by the organism's defences.

It is only in the third phase with the appearance of metastases, of dissemination, that the organism starts to give up the struggle. Nevertheless, even at this stage, it still possesses resources which therapy can turn to account.

The duration of the evolution of cancer varies above all with age. In the young, in whom the processes of growth are still fully active, the condition proceeds apace, to such an extent that it becomes difficult to distinguish between the stages. In the elderly, on the contrary, any possibility of regeneration has been lost, and one observes that the stages are sometimes so drawn out that the cancer is not the actual cause of death.

In the light of what has been said above, the aim of the treatment of cancer will be to re-establish equilibrium between the structural forces and the forces of proliferation. We have three essential objects: (1) reinforcement of the organism's defences and form-giving powers; (2) promoting metamorphosis of the vegetative forces; (3) preservation of the organism from harmful external effects.

Does orthodox treatment attain these objectives? Neither surgery, radium, X-rays nor cytostatic drugs can claim to do so. They do not strengthen formative, structural forces and have no action on metamorphosis of the etheric forces. X-ray treatment, like surgery, aims at destroying the tumour, which is only a local symptom of the cancer condition. Both considerably weaken the organism's defences, and also often lead to relapses and the worsening of the patient's general condition. Is that to say that they must be entirely rejected? It is certain that the tumour, living at the expense of the organism, constitutes in itself an enfeebling and intoxicating factor which it is valuable to be rid of. Surgery, when possible and on condition that it is limited to minimal intervention, seems preferable to treatment by radium or X-rays which leave the organism the trouble of eliminating residues resulting from tissue destruction. As for cytostatic drugs, these obstruct cell proliferation in a non-selective manner, reducing it in the tumour whose destruction is wished for, just as much as where it is essential to life—hence their harmful secondary

effects. There remain the hormones. Their action is much
more selective; their use has specific effects on proliferating
cancer cells, but undesirable effects on the whole organism.
This may present disadvantages as one knows and one cannot
therefore, properly speaking, attribute a curative action to
them.

Does any remedy exist which is capable of attaining the
first objective, that of strengthening the defences of the
organism in the direction of enhancing structural form?
Rudolf Steiner suggested the use of mistletoe (*Viscum album*)
to doctors who asked his advice. This plant, known from very
ancient times to possess certain therapeutic virtues, had never
before been used in the treatment of cancer. Steiner gave
indications on numerous occasions for both the preparation
and the use of mistletoe.

Why mistletoe? The first thing that strikes us when we
observe this plant is its spherical form. We do not find in it, as
in plants growing in the soil, that differentiation between
upper and lower parts, between forces of gravity and of
lightness. Whatever may be the site of attachment of its
sucker, mistletoe grows perpendicularly to the branch which
bears it, in accordance with its own laws and its own rhythm,
and freed from the conditions to which other plants must
submit. It remains green the whole year long, independently
of its exposure to light. Even its sucker stores up chlorophyll
in the darkness of the wood in which it has buried itself. The
berries of the mistletoe ripen in winter, doing so without
warmth. The leaves themselves are indifferent to light-
orientation. Thus mistletoe is neither geotropic nor photo-
tropic, and has freed itself from both solar and terrestrial
forces equally; this confers on it a very special place in the
vegetable kingdom. It is in a way an anachronistic plant
which has remained behind from the earth's evolutionary
past. That is why it cannot grow directly in the soil and needs

an intermediate host. We could say that it repulses the terrestrial forces, and thus behaves in a manner which is the opposite to that of a tumour which opens itself to them. Steiner has also said that mistletoe resists the action of the etheric forces, i.e. proliferative forces. These properties have been confirmed by pharmacodynamic research.

Steiner has given many other suggestions regarding mistletoe's properties against cancer. We cannot enter into them here, for their understanding presupposes a deep knowledge of anthroposophy. It must, however, be pointed out that Steiner insisted that it was necessary for the mistletoe to undergo processing to make it into a true remedy for cancer by strengthening this characteristic of emancipation from cosmic and terrestrial forces of which we have spoken.

Shouldering this task, Kaelin in 1928 and, from 1934 onwards, his co-worker Leroi (1906–68) worked on developing this remedy, to which Steiner gave the name Iscador. In 1949 Leroi founded the institute Hiscia at Arlesheim (Switzerland) where he pursued his cancer research together with his wife, Dr R. Leroi von May. The Lukas Clinic, adjacent to Hiscia, specializes in the post-operative treatment of cancer.

The preparation of mistletoe and its method of use have thus been steadily developed. In contrast to cytostatic drugs, Iscador does not cause blood disorders and its use can be continued for many years without any disadvantages. It does not act in a non-specific manner, but concentrates its action in the area round the tumour where it causes hyperaemia and a rise in temperature. This reaction makes it necessary for a certain caution to be exercised in the treatment of cerebral tumours because of the increased intracranial pressure it might possibly provoke.

Iscador is capable of being improved further.[11] It has not yet attained the aim that Rudolf Steiner set for it—to replace the scalpel. Nevertheless it is at the present moment the sole remedy capable of strengthening the defences of the organism in its preservation of form. Thus patients who have radiation treatment have been able to withstand much higher doses of X-rays when they have received injections of Iscador at the same time. Comparative researches carried out over several years in different European clinics have shown the superiority of Iscador over all other treatments.

The second objective, to achieve correct metamorphosis of the etheric forces, cannot be achieved through medicines. One may even ask whether it is at all possible to accomplish this, the moment having passed when it should normally have been achieved. It is certainly unlikely that what should have been transformed during the first seven years of life can then be attained retrospectively during adult life. It is certainly possible to give help through various curative artistic activities such as painting, modelling and curative eurythmy. The systematic use of these artistic therapies at the Lukas Clinic is certainly a factor which brings about significant improvement in this direction.

The psychological state is of the very greatest importance in cancer. We have seen that it can be an agitating cause of the condition. A complete cure is only really possible inasmuch as we transform the patient 'internally'. Therapeutic artistic activities can be a big step in the direction of spiritualization, and therefore of metamorphosis of forces to a higher level. The patient's participation in his treatment is essential, and this is only possible if he knows what is wrong with him. We have no right to leave a patient in a limbo of uncertainty. Much tact is required in telling him the diagnosis and especially in showing him that his condition is not incurable.

Rightly handled, the patient can then find courage and take an active part in the fight against his illness. This point of view is not of theoretical importance only. Personally I have always had better results with patients who knew what their disease was. A patient who has been told this knows that his doctor is not lying to him, and this gives him confidence in the physician and helps him to fight his illness. This creates a vastly different milieu from that dreadful atmosphere of false compassion, when the patient is surrounded by a tissue of lies, which he confronts with silent unbelief.

Treatment of cancer requires the mobilization of all the forces at our disposal. We associate different complementary treatments with Iscador, and we pay particular attention to treatment of the liver. Caspar Blond[12] has shown the prominent part played by this organ in cancer.

We must also consider the third objective of treatment: the preservation of the organism from harmful external actions. This usually necessitates a change in the mode of life, the creation of a favourable environment and above all a healthy diet. This often poses problems which are today almost insoluble. How can one, for example, obtain products of high quality which have not been denatured? How can one be sure of their true value? The presence of harmful substances, pesticides for example, can, up to a point, be revealed by chemical analysis. Quality could be checked with the help of sensitive crystallization, but these methods are not within the reach of ordinary people. Health food shops seldom provide satisfactory warranties for their produce and I have seen vegetables that had been refused by one group of shops, because analysis had revealed the presence of pesticides, being offered for sale and recommended by a competitor! If one cannot have a garden of one's own, the only possibility is to know the producer personally and assess his integrity. One must also train oneself to recognize what has been grown in a healthy manner by its appearance and taste. Vegetables grown by biodynamic methods of cultivation are ideal.[13]

Treatment of malignant tumours by Iscador sometimes

gives unexpectedly good results. Nevertheless it is preferable to treat patients early in the pre-cancerous stage of the condition, in which phase success is almost certain. It will be objected that it is difficult to judge the efficacy of treatment in the absence of a tumour, but that is incorrect. In the first place improvement in the general condition of the patient gives some indication. It is also possible to check the evolution of the disease by examination of the blood through sensitive crystallization or the capillary-dynamic method. Finally, patients in whom a pre-cancerous condition has been diagnosed sometimes do not, for various reasons, keep to their treatment, and several years later become subjects of confirmed malignant tumours. That is obviously a proof that one would prefer to do without!

In the prophylaxis of this condition what has been said about environment, manner of life and food must not be neglected; but cancer prevention also includes one other essential factor. If we wish to work on the process of metamorphosis of the etheric forces into thought forces, this must be carried out at the time when this normally occurs, i.e. during the school years. Neither can we emphasize too strongly the part played by the teacher in allowing the child to develop harmoniously. It is essential that such teaching should take into account what we have described in the second part of this work.

15
THE MENSTRUAL CYCLE

Observation of the menstrual cycle leads us to divide it into two main phases, the first characterized by growth of the endometrium and the second by degeneration of the endometrium and the elimination of the products of this breakdown. Such processes, as we have seen in Chapter 2, are the expression of the action of the ego and also of the astral body, first working with the etheric body in the lower pole of the organism, then working more directly from the upper pole. The alternation of these two phases constitutes the rhythm proper to the whole of the female generative organs.

The part played by the ego is equally expressed in the fact that the menstrual function is in close association with the blood—the organ of the ego—and with haemopoiesis. The role of the ego is also clear from the fact that menstruation is an exclusively human process which is not found in animals. Phenomena enabling procreation to occur in animals generally follow an annual rhythm, that is to say a rhythm similar to that of plants which we can therefore regard as etheric in nature. Animals have no menstrual periods and even the pseudo-menstruation of *Macacus rhesus* monkeys is anovular. Finally, the fact that a rise in temperature can sometimes take the place of a menstruation points to a relationship with the action of the ego.

Just as we have related the rhythm of the heart to that of the sun, so are we led to compare the twenty-eight-day periodicity of the menstrual cycle with that of the phases of the moon. We know, however, that menstruation is not totally determined by the moon, for otherwise all women would have their periods at the same time. The lunar rhythm has clearly been interiorized into the female organism and in menstruation we see a reminder of this.

Looking at the phenomenon from a purely materialistic point of view might well give rise to the objection that the succession of the two phases of the cycle is purely automatic, each process leading to the following one, just as a pendulum starts its downward course when it has reached a certain height. However, the fact that a longer cycle will usually follow a cycle that has been shortened due to external circumstances, or vice versa, shows the existence of a process of inner compensation, and therefore of internal regulation which we can only modify temporarily. It is this capacity which demonstrates that the menstrual cycle is not a mere mechanism. If we put a clock out of adjustment, it maintains its deviation as long as we do not adjust it accurately again. If, on the other hand, we disturb the menstrual cycle by means of a hormone injection, the organism has the tendency to compensate for the deviation by itself, so as to find its own natural rhythm again. It is of course possible to disturb the organism to such a degree that it becomes impossible for it to readjust itself. But the possibility of destroying a function within an organism is very far from being proof of its non-existence.

The first phase of the cycle, which lasts from the end of menstruation to ovulation on the fourteenth day, is characterized by this action of the ego, modified through the mediation successively of the astral body, the etheric body and the physical body. These confer on the reproductive organs that motive force proper to the metabolic pole, which is characterized by processes of proliferation, synthesis and elaboration. At the level of the ovary this motive force shows itself by maturation of the ovum and the formation of the Graafian follicle, and at the level of the uterus by proliferation of the endometrium in preparation for the embedding of the ovum. This proliferative phase extends even a little beyond the time of ovulation, for the formation of the corpus luteum is also part of it. If the ovum is fertilized, this corpus luteum persists throughout pregnancy. This constitutes a prolongation and reinforcement of this first phase. The unfertilized ovum, on the other hand, dies and this is the first step of the second phase which is characterized by the direct action of the ego on the organism, which induces processes of degeneration. The corpus luteum then withers, leaving a small fibrous nodule. The uterine mucous membrane degenerates and becomes congested with blood and loses its vitality, and will be eliminated at the time of menstruation. This excretion of now lifeless material is accompanied by contractions of the uterus, which is evidence of an increased activity of the astral body.

In reality the passage of the first into the second phase is not so clear-cut as our rather schematic description might lead one to suppose. Thus ovulation is an excretory process, necessitating the intervention of the astral body. It really heralds the second phase, although taking place towards the end of the first. The formation of the corpus luteum, on the other hand, is a proliferative process, belonging to the first phase although overlapping into the second. The formation of the hormones, folliculin and lutein, is evidence of a glandular activity arising from the etheric body and belonging to the first phase; but the excretion of these hormones into the circulation is a process of elimination proper to the second. This demonstrates that within the organism the actual substances are of less moment than the processes from which they arise.

These two hormones, folliculin and lutein, continue to be secreted throughout pregnancy. Their formation therefore is truly part of the processes of elaboration and, in the absence of pregnancy, they are connected with the first phase of the menstrual cycle.

This sketch of the menstrual cycle in relation to the constituent elements of the human being is indispensable to understanding menstrual disorders, and will also allow us to establish a rational treatment for them. We see at once the possibility of two anomalies, one characterized by excess of the processes of elaboration and proliferation, and the other by an excess of those of degeneration.

When the proliferative tendency gains the upper hand, this shows itself in glandular hyperplasia, hypertrophy of the mucous membrane, and an excess of folliculin. The hyperaemia which accompanies the first phase continues during the second, and menstrual flow increases. The blood which is eliminated is bright red, incompletely broken down and retains an arterial character. The bleeding is not, as in normal menstruation, the result of degeneration of the mucous membrane, but a result of its congestion. It is like an explosion, and the flow is usually early. These disturbances are often accompanied by giddiness, fainting, inattention and a tendency to forgetfulness which are characteristic of a diminution of consciousness. These patients, often plethoric, have a tendency to migraine (cf. p. 37). This is the *Calcarea carbonica* type of the homoeopaths. In this type of patient, what corresponds to the soft living substance of the oyster predominates over the dead mineral substance of the shell.

When the tendencies of the second phase predominate, and degeneration, disintegration and death take the upper hand, we observe phenomena of stasis which are not limited to the uterine mucous membrane. The veins dilate and the extremities are cyanosed. The scanty dark menses appear late. Here we have the *Pulsatilla* type of the homoeopaths. These are patients in whom the earth forces—gravity, for example—predominate. The venous stagnation is an expression of the force of gravity. The tendency to melancholy, the mental slowness and the head bent forwards towards the earth are other signs. The pasque flower (*Pulsatilla vulgaris*) is characterized by a strong taproot highly imbued with earth forces. The leaves, in contrast, are finely divided and open themselves widely to cosmic forces; and then the bell-shaped flower is bent towards the earth, and is subject in its turn to the forces of gravity. Finally, on ripening, the stem becomes straight again and the seeds with their long silky plumes turn once more towards the cosmos. The whole plant is thus the rhythmic expression of a conflict between terrestrial and cosmic forces which ends in the victory of the latter. Death and resurrection are concentrated in this pasque flower. The preference of this plant for siliceous soils reminds us of the polarity between *Calcarea carbonica* and *Pulsatilla*.

When the forces of the ego are called upon too strongly at the upper pole—which happens frequently at times of excessive mental activity such as occur during study and preparation for exams—these forces are no longer available to the lower pole for the generative functions. Moreover, the intense breaking-down processes which excessive mental activity entails have to be compensated for unceasingly by etheric forces of regeneration. This reduction of both the forces of the ego and of those of the etheric body at the lower pole makes the processes of maturation of the ovum and of proliferation of the uterine mucous membrane impossible. The first phase of the cycle is suppressed and, as the second cannot take place without the preparation constituted by the first, the menstrual cycle and menstruation no longer take place. We are then faced with amenorrhoea from a diminution of these forces. Associated with the general process there is often a factor which triggers this condition—sudden chilling from bathing or mental shock, for example.

As long as the cause, i.e. excessive mental activity, persists, cure is not possible. The patient's way of life must first be changed. But cure is difficult. The ego, which should be the actor at the lower pole, behaves more like a spectator at the upper pole and, once installed in its seat, has no great wish to come down onto the stage again and take up its role once more. Sometimes 'tricks' have to be used to get it to come down. One of these is warming the lower pole, for heat is the element of the ego.

The amenorrhoea of young anaemic girls is rather different. We do not find mental overactivity in this case. The ego incarnates reluctantly, just as much at the superior pole as at the inferior. To revert to the previous picture, we say that it no more likes its seat in the dress circle than its place on the stage, and is reluctant to enter the theatre at all. This type of amenorrhoea calls primarily for treatment of the anaemia (cf. pp. 100–01). It must be added that this type of amenorrhoea and the preceding one are sometimes found together in the same patient.

Normally the reproductive organs undergo a transformation during the second seven-year period of life under the influence of the astral body. If the astral body does not play its part correctly, these organs do not reach maturity and remain infantile, so that the secondary sexual characteristics—hair and breast development, change in the voice, etc.—do not appear. Metamorphosis of the etheric forces on the functional plane does not take place, with the natural consequence that etheric organs such as the thymus remain inactive. Such is the position in primary amenorrhoea.

Besides secondary amenorrhoea due to withdrawal of forces as described above, there exists also a type which in contrast reflects overactivity of the etheric body, which hypertrophies and becomes in a way 'impermeable' to the action of the astral body and the ego, which cannot then assume their functions of differentiation. Ovulation does not, therefore, occur, and the process of degeneration is even more inhibited, and consequently the second phase is also absent.

The processes of growth, which should limit themselves to the uterine endometrium, then have a tendency to invade the whole organism, causing obesity and fluid retention in the tissues. This resembles, to some degree, what happens in pregnancy, and it is not uncommon to see this form of amenorrhoea following pregnancy.

By mentioning *Calc. carb.* and *Pulsatilla* we have pointed the way to treatment. Generally speaking, we use the calcareous substance when the processes of the first phase are excessive and have a tendency to overstep their bounds; and we use *Pulsatilla* in patients when those of the second phase are too intense. When there is a tendency to menorrhagia, Rudolf Steiner advised the use of *Corallium rubrum* in preference to *Calc.* It is prescribed in triturition in 3x, or better still in the form of daily inunctions in the suprapubic region (*Ungt. Corallium rubrum* comp.). When there is severe haemorrhage we may resort to one or more suprapubic injections of *Marmor* 6x/*Stibium* 6x aa. We also obtain excellent results with that very modest plant shepherd's purse—*Capsella bursa pastoris* 10% to 3x by mouth.

When the breaking-down processes of the second phase are too predominant and the terrestrial forces get the upper hand, we give *Pulsatilla* 3x–6x, i.e. in the presence of venous stasis and a disposition to melancholy. It is equally necessary to strengthen the action of the etheric body by prescribing *Argentum* which it is especially beneficial to apply at night in the form of an ointment (*Ungt. argenti* 0.4%) over the suprapubic region. These applications are made during the first phase of the cycle, alternating with the administration of *Pulsatilla* during the second phase. *Prunus spinosa* 3x–5x is prescribed as a supplementary remedy.

In practice we often come across cases of menstrual disorders which it may be difficult to classify under one or other of the tendencies described above and which are generally grouped under the term dysmenorrhoea. These disorders are the expression of a lack of harmony between the different constitutional elements. They are often accompanied by spasmodic phenomena in relation to the astral body, and consequently appear at times in the cycle when the astral body normally comes into play. Thus the menses, which represent an excretion of residues from the breaking down of the mucous membrane engorged with blood, are accompanied at the end of the second phase by uterine contractions incited by the astral body. These contractions can assume a spasmodic character, which manifests as painful cramps. A disorder of the same nature appears, though in a less severe degree, at the time of ovulation, which is also a process of excretion involving the participation of the astral body.

Disorders of a spastic character are relieved by prescribing *Chamomilla* 20x/*Tormentilla* 30x, ten drops three times a day before meals, the treatment to be started two days before the expected onset of menstruation and continued as long as necessary. We can also use *Belladonna* 6x (for brunettes) or *Chamomilla* 3x (for blondes). This treatment by mouth is complemented if necessary by daily suprapubic inunctions with *Ungt. Oxalis* 10% (or even 30%). The application of *Ungt. Cupri* 0.4% in the lumbar region should also be considered.

True cure of dysmenorrhoea nevertheless calls for treatment in greater depth. As this condition is often due to chronic chilling of the lower extremities, no cure is possible unless the patient can be persuaded to wear adequate clothing. You will often find the legs of these patients icy to the touch, although they declare they do not feel cold. Treatment in depth, applicable to all menstrual troubles, is achieved by Menodoron, whose composition we owe to Rudolf Steiner (*Achillea millefolium,* herb 4%/*Capsella bursa pastoris,* herb 3%/*Origanum majorana* seeds 6%/*Quercus robur* bark 5%/

Urtica dioica, flowers 2%). Five to ten drops are given three times a day before meals. This treatment must be pursued for several months, being interrupted during the menstrual period. It can be accompanied, or followed, by a course of treatment with Metra Tea (an infusion at bedtime). Menodoron and Metra Tea have, through their harmonizing action, an effect on all menstrual disorders, whatever their origin.

Treatment of amenorrhoea often presents a more difficult problem, especially primary amenorrhoea which may well require the use of constitutional remedies. In order to encourage the ego to come down again to the reproductive sphere and to carry out its function there, we prescribe *Levisticum* 6x, alternately with *Ovaria* 3x, each in a dose of ten drops twice daily (one can also mix them together instead of giving them alternately). Along the same lines we can prescribe *Phosphorus* 6x, ten drops on waking. We can also prescribe *Conchae* or *Pulsatilla* according to the type of illness we have to deal with. When the menses start again, a course of treatment with Menodoron and Metra Tea should be started and continued over a long period.

16
DISEASES OF THE SKIN

Works on dermatology impress one by the minutiae of their descriptions and the attention to detail to which the microscope has largely contributed. But they barely come to grips with the real problem, the cause of these cutaneous conditions. Treatment, disappointingly, is frequently limited to palliative measures. Study of some skin conditions will demonstrate that it is possible to understand the genesis of these illnesses more fully by examining their relationship to the totality of the human organism, and this then opens the way for a more rational therapy.

In the skin we find reflected the human being's threefold nature, that is, a nerve-sense pole, a metabolic pole and a mediating rhythmic part. This threefold quality is apparent as much on the anatomical plane as on the functional.

Inasmuch as it is a sense organ, the skin obviously belongs to the nerve-sense system. But it also possesses another characteristic proper to the cephalic pole—that of shaping the organism. It confines the physical body within limits and we owe our external form to it. It brings into opposition the sculpturing or shaping forces of an astral nature, which act centripetally, and the etheric forces of growth, which act centrifugally. It is in the balance between these forces, both of which have received the imprint of the ego, that the beauty of forms such as we can admire in the Aphrodite of Cnidos resides. The centrifugal forces which are dominant in the child have the tendency to fill out, round off or even swell out the bodily forms, while in the old person, on the other hand, the sculpturing and mineralizing forces have the upper hand, so that distension due to the centrifugal forces disappears. The skin loses its elasticity and becomes flaccid. Wrinkles appear like hinges between areas of more rigid skin. This constitutes a process similar to, though less marked than, the articulation between the different elements of the shells of invertebrates. We see, in fact, the tendency as we grow old to become, physically, invertebrates. As a counterpoise to this process we ought, with age, to strengthen our moral character, to become 'vertebrates' on an ethical level and not be satisfied merely with the support which we can obtain from the carapace of social or religious conventions.

In animals, even apart from invertebrates, the hard elements of the skin—fur, feathers, scales, horns, hoofs, etc.—are much more developed than in man. For man has metamorphosed into powers of thinking those forces which are necessary for the growth of these elements (cf. p. 88). So it is that man must clothe himself. The awareness of his nakedness, after tasting the fruit of the tree of knowledge, is symptomatic of human nature as distinct from animal nature.

The structure of the outer layer of the epidermis, composed of dead cells, is a typical example of the dying and mineralizing tendency of the nerve-sense pole. Its translucency recalls the appearance of silica which is also found in relatively high quantities in the skin, hair and nails. This translucency, which diminishes with pigmentation, enables us to understand what happens in the vascular layer of the dermis, the rhythmic region of the skin. Emotions or soul activities are accompanied by circulatory changes which cause reddening or paleness of the skin. The rhythmic manifestations of the skin are expressed by its respiratory-like function, whose importance we are all aware of.

Finally we find a number of metabolic processes in the skin, localized principally in the hypodermis, the deepest layer. The sweat glands are situated in this layer, as are the hair follicles which are sites of marked proliferative activity. In some regions—the face for example—the skin also possesses a delicate musculature whose activity is revealed in mimicry.

The skin thus has a relationship with all three divisions—nerve-sense, rhythmic and metabolic—within the organism of which it is the reflection. Skin conditions are thus often the result of disturbances in these regions. The participation of the skin in these disturbances is generally an expression of the exteriorization of morbid processes, which constitute an attempt at healing. The frequent appearance of asthma after suppression of an exudative diathesis and its disappearance when the skin symptoms reappear is evidence of this. This type of illness is the result of an incomplete transformation of protein. The skin tries to transform and eliminate what has not been properly metabolized by the internal organs. This hypertrophy of the metabolic functions of the skin is accompanied by centrifugal manifestations through the skin. Erythema, papules and vesicles are but different degrees of a process of 'digestion' or excretion of foreign proteins. We find these symptoms again in different degrees in pyoderma, furunculosis, weeping eczema, etc. These are manifestations of youthful skin and this is why one finds them more often at the beginning than at the end of life.

When the processes of devitalization and mineralization become excessively strong, we find the dry dermatoses—ichthyosis, psoriasis, dry eczema, etc. This group also includes itchy conditions whose severity is often in contrast with a poverty of or absence of objective signs, for pruritis is a hypertrophy of the nerve-sense processes which causes scratching. This last may constitute an attempt to eliminate elements that are too hard, scabs for example.

Some skin conditions seem to belong at the same time to both metabolic and nerve-sense processes. Such is the case in urticaria, of which the eruption is a metabolic symptom and the itching a nerve-sense manifestation. This double relationship really points to a disturbance of the rhythmic system of the skin in its circulatory aspect. Other conditions related to this system have rather a 'respiratory' character. Generally speaking, this very important function of the skin and its repercussions on the organism are far too neglected by medicine. The mycoses probably result from respiratory disturbances of the skin reacting at the dermatological level. Fungi can generally develop only in a poorly oxygenated environment, so that one often finds the use of poor quality cosmetics or synthetic detergents associated with the development of mycotic conditions. Thus the appearance on the market of certain detergents has been accompanied by veritable epidemics of paronychia among housewives. Deodorants and antiperspirants which hinder sweat secretion give rise to true processes of autointoxication comparable with that caused by retention of urine. It is important to know that unpleasant perspiratory odours are sometimes due to changes in the sweat brought about by bacteria, helped by the alkalinity of soaps or by the wearing of synthetic textiles. In other cases the odour of the perspiration has a dietary origin.

A certain number of skin diseases, such as warts and papillomata, cannot be included in any of the preceding categories. The cause of these is a localized defect in the restraining function of the skin. It is as if there were a hole in the skin through which the proliferative processes had escaped. There really is an 'etheric hole', a small area where the human etheric is absent, allowing viruses to insinuate themselves and to develop their own etheric and to proliferate. This process presents a certain resemblance to that which we have described in cancer (cf. pp. 163–4). This local weakness of the human etheric is related to its intensification in another region in connection with a deeper disorder. If this deeper disorder is remedied then the etheric will resume its place and the cutaneous manifestations will disappear.

The existence of internal disorders in relation to peripheral manifestations, such as the skin diseases, is almost invariable; and even in those which appear to be due solely to external agencies there is often a predisposing and underlying factor. This explains why certain people are more resistant than others to these agencies. These deep disturbances often relate to the functions of the liver, for a polarity exists between the liver and the skin.

The soft indefinite shape of the liver is in contrast with the structured nature of the skin with its hard elements—the horny layer, hair and nails. The predominance of the liquid element in the liver contrasts with the dryness and mineralization of the skin. If the liver is the warm pole of the organism, the skin is, on the contrary, the coldest region. The liver is a predominantly venous organ, while the rose-red colour of the skin is the expression of the presence of arterial blood. We can easily understand this when this characteristic disappears, as in cyanosis. Finally the insensibility of the liver, a metabolic organ, is in contrast with the extreme sensitivity of the skin, a principally nerve-sense organ. Nevertheless the two organs do possess one property in common—their strong powers of regeneration. Side by side with this, in the skin there is a no less intense process of devitalization of the epidermal cells, hair and nails.

When certain hepatic functions are deficient, the skin has a tendency to substitute itself for them. The skin then becomes warmer, moister and less sensitive, and loses its shape, giving rise to papules, vesicles, etc., and the polarity between the two organs is lessened. We observe processes such as these in the exudative diatheses.

Treatment of these dermatoses therefore calls especially for the institution of a diet to relieve the liver and for basic liver treatment (cf. Chapter 11). To this we may add a more specialized therapy.

Starting with birch (cf. p. 66), we have seen that this plant has the property of dividing up the processes of protein formation and of mineralization, the former directed towards the leaf and the latter towards the bark. With the extract of birch leaves we help the organism to assume its processes of protein formation correctly and at the appropriate site. By this means one can avoid their displacement towards the skin. Thus we prescribe *Betula fol.* 3x, ten drops three times a day before meals.

Sulphur is necessary for the metabolism of proteins, and we prescribe it in the form of *Sulphur* 3x–6x. This often provokes a short-lived exacerbation of the symptoms, which does not constitute a contra-indication for its use. We can also associate sulphur with iron when the respiratory function of the skin appears to be hindered. We then prescribe *Ferrum sulphid. nat.* (pyrites) 3x trit. When the sulphur in the organism appears to want to escape from living processes, which shows itself by the unpleasant odour of the secretions, we prescribe *Hepar sulphuris calcareum* 4x–6x. We can also have recourse to the structure promoting forces of antimony, in the form of *Stibium praep.* 6x–10x.

In plethoric patients who give the impression of flabbiness and ill-defined outlines we use oyster shell—*Conchae* in medium or high dilution (15x–30x).

The temptation to apply external treatment to these dermatoses is strong, in that the patient always has the impression that he is not being properly cared for if we do not directly attack the visible symptoms. It is not always easy to make him understand the internal origin of his condition. One must never forget, however, that the abrupt suppression of discharges can become the cause of much more serious disturbances. One is satisfied, therefore, with hygienic measures consisting of bathing with baths of warm water to which *Calendula* 20% has been added—one or two tea-spoonfuls are enough for a bath—or better still an infusion of *Species eczema* (Eczema Tea). The latter is also administered by mouth—one or two cups a day. Soaps, detergents and all kinds of skin creams are forbidden.

We have seen (Chapter 3) that the direct action of the ego on the organism, such as is manifested principally at the upper pole, causes devitalization and mineralization. But the ego possesses, on the other hand, the ability to overcome these minerals and to 'crush' them. The processes of de-vitalization are necessary for the existence of awakened consciousness, but demineralization, on the contrary, is inti-mately bound up with the awareness we have of ourselves as individuals. But the ego is limited in its ability to demin-eralize. If devitalization and breaking down are excessive in relation to the possibilities of the ego, residues and deposits are formed which behave like foreign bodies.

We find these processes of demineralization and elimin-ation of salts again in the human skin. Given its principally nerve-sense character, this does not surprise us. When these processes of demineralization are insufficient in relation to those of the contrary tendency, the hard elements accumulate, making the skin dry, scabby or scaly as we find in ichthyosis, dry eczema and psoriasis. To a certain degree it takes on an animal character, which is particularly marked in ichthyosis. There is, therefore, a relationship between the character of our skin, which contains much less of the horny elements than that of animals, and the consciousness of self, which belongs to the human race alone.

We use birch bark in order to arrest the course of these indurated conditions of the skin. This favours orientation towards the periphery and stimulates the elimination of what has become too hard and too mineral. We prescribe *Betula cortex* 1% by subcutaneous injection or by mouth. This does not prevent us giving birch leaves at the same time for their vitalizing and diuretic properties, for example in the form of Birch Elixir.

We also awaken the demineralizing forces of the ego by the administration of a hard mineral such as silica. We therefore prescribe it in small doses, in medium or high dilution—*Quartz* 15x–30x. trit., a teaspoon once or twice a week. We direct its action towards the skin by associating it with *Betula cort.*

As a general prophylaxis, we strengthen the ego in its task of demineralization by means of rosemary. This should be brought into contact with the skin in a finely dispersed form. With this in view we employ Rosemary Bath Milk or Rosemary Massage Oil. Their use in the morning awakens consciousness and, through this effect, assists in securing sound sleep; however, for the same reason their use at night may cause insomnia. We have yet another excellent means of combating hardening of the skin—sulphur baths (*Kalium sulph.* 30%, one dessertspoonful for a bath).

We employ very hot bathing with the infusion of *Species eczema* for conditions with much itching. The more severe the itching, the hotter the water used for bathing the affected part! The infusion can equally be added to a hot bath when the lesions are extensive. In senile pruritis, which is always associated with arteriosclerosis, one must not forget to prescribe *Plumbum melit.* and Birch Elixir (cf. pp. 67–8).

In psoriasis we obtain good results by starting treatment with an apple diet for one week, followed by three months on a vegetarian diet. Subsequently the patient abstains from all fats of animal origin. In addition to *Betula cortex* and *Quartz*, we prescribe *Gallae halepenses* 2x–3x trit., a salt-spoonful three times a day, and *Agaricus muscarius* 10x, ten drops twice a day in a decoction of *Species antipsoriases*. In severe cases injections of *Formica* 6x–15x are given twice weekly.

Juvenile acne is characterized by the retention of sebum and debris, which forms the comodone. The skin reacts to this as to a foreign body and produces an inflammatory and eliminative reaction, the whole constituting the acne pimple. It originates, therefore, in a defect in the processes of excretion. In young girls it often accompanies the first phase of the menstrual cycle and an excess of folliculin (cf. Chapter 15). When acne is localized especially on the chest in the tall, thin type of patient, one must think of the possibility of a predisposition to tuberculosis. We are, therefore, not too assiduous in curing the furunculosis as such, but attend particularly to the general state of health.

The treatment of acne calls for a diet resembling that recommended for psoriasis—one week apple diet and three months vegetarian diet. In addition to this general treatment *Quartz* 30x (replaced in certain patients by *Conchae*) is given alternately with *Sulphur* 3x. One has recourse to Erysidoron 1 and 2 in severe cases. Constipation must also be dealt with, for example by drinking a weak infusion of Clairo Tea at bedtime. The excretory functions of the astral body must always be stimulated, especially through sweating. Washing with, and the application of compresses of, water *as hot as possible*, to which one or two teaspoonfuls of *Calendula* 20% are added, is carried out locally both morning and evening.

One prefers to abstain from the application of any ointment except in the case of indurated acne, when *Mercurius vivus* 15x ointment may be employed. Let us note that this ointment gives equally good results with induration in other situations, such as chalazion. This ointment is applied at night after bathing with *Calendula*. Sea bathing and sunbathing, practised in moderation, are helpful in the treatment of acne.

Fungal infections of the skin are also treated by very hot bathing with *Calendula* night and morning. After the morning bathing W.C.S. Powder (Silica 0.1%/Antimony 0.1%/*Arnica* 2%/*Calendula* 3.3%/*Echinacea* 1%) is applied, and after the evening bathing a little *Cupri* 0.4%/*Nicotiana* 1% as an ointment. When there is intertrigo, a little gauze or cotton wool is placed between the skin folds to help aerate them. Fungal infections are exacerbated by alkaline soaps and the use of these should be avoided. An acid soap should be used instead, and clothes that come into contact with the affected parts should be given an acid rinse with water to which a little vinegar or lemon juice has been added. These precautions apply equally to bromidosis and can often eliminate this condition.

Although not actually 'diseases' of the skin but the result of trauma, it is important to deal at this point with wounds and burns, for their eventual results depend very much on the nature of their early treatment.

Wounds are washed with warm water to which *Calendula* 20% has been added in the proportion of one teaspoonful to a bowl of water. If necessary one cleans up the wound and leaves on it a compress of the diluted *Calendula*. NB: It must never be used undiluted. When healing starts, *Calendula/ Mercurialis* comp. ointment may be used instead of the compresses. When there is a tendency to infection the warm water for the bathing and compresses is replaced by hot. Healing of wounds treated in this manner is remarkable. If the wound is a linear one, in other words a cut, after careful washing the edges of the wound may be drawn together with transparent adhesive tape and sutures are thus avoided. When the wound is deep, such as one caused by a nail, a very hot Calendula bath is given. If an antitetanus prophylaxis appears necessary, a subcutaneous injection of *Belladonna* 15x/*Hyoscyamus* 30x aa is given.

Burns are treated by compresses of Combudoron (*Arnica pl. tot.* 2.5%/*Urtica urens herba* 47.5%). A freshly prepared solution is made by adding one dessertspoonful of Combudoron to nine dessertspoonfuls of water and the compresses are soaked in this. These should be left in place and periodically moistened. They must never be allowed to dry. The compresses may be removed after five days and renewed if necessary or, if epithelialization is complete, replaced by Combudoron ointment. The period of five days may be considerably shortened in small superficial burns. This treatment of burns is remarkable for the rapidity of the relief which usually appears after a quarter of an hour, for the rapidity of healing and for the excellent cicatrization which does not result in any cheloid formation. In cases of extensive burns general treatment of the patient must also be given— *Arnica pl. tot. 3x*, ten drops three to six times in twenty-four hours, Cardiodoron ten drops three times a day, *Argentun* 30x one subcutaneous injection every one or two days, and drinking of much water to which Birch Elixir has been added to encourage diuresis. Combudoron also gives relief and rapid healing in arc flashes (diluted 1 in 20 and applied as a compress to the closed eyelids) and in sunburn (to be treated like burns).

The anthroposophical pharmacopoeia includes a number of ointments but few of them are intended for treatment of skin conditions. By the oral administration of a remedy one calls principally on the metabolism; subcutaneous administration brings the rhythmic system into play; while the application of a remedy in the form of an ointment to the sense organ, which the skin is, makes an appeal especially to the nerve-sense system. The remedy applied does not work by its actual penetration through the skin but by its dynamic action. It is also possible to assimilate a potentized medicament applied in the form of an ointment. The demonstrable efficacy of this form of therapy is a striking proof that the modern sciences have not yet been able to offer us all the answers in relation to the phenomena of life.

POSTSCRIPT

When you opened this book, dear reader, you would have been seeking the answers to many questions. If I have been able to elucidate some, I shall certainly have raised many others.

I have dealt only with a limited number of conditions in these pages and am far from having called upon all Rudolf Steiner's medical ideas and suggestions. But I shall perhaps have better fulfilled my aim by arousing your curiosity than by propounding blindly applicable remedies.

Some ideas will have seemed unusual to you on first reading, for it is difficult to grasp them by intellectual thinking alone, and the pictures which I have happened to use will perhaps have made you smile.

Put this book on one side for a while. Then when you take it up again, you may find that you see things in a new light, and what may have seemed preposterous at first sight will now appear helpful.

It is in practising anthroposophical medicine that these ideas and approaches will show their worth; for anthroposophy is a path which it is not enough to follow on a map but which demands to be practised. It is a path of development, a transformation of the self.

NOTE ON THE PHARMACEUTICAL
PREPARATIONS

The remedies proposed by Rudolf Steiner are not simple mixtures. In order that the natural substance may become a remedy it is necessary for it to undergo certain methods of preparation of which Steiner gave the main outlines, leaving to his pupils the task of working them out in detail. A laboratory was set up in Arlesheim, Switzerland, for this purpose, directed towards both research and production. Steiner gave it the name of Weleda. Associated laboratories have come into being throughout the world. Research on the efficacy of preparations, optimum time for harvesting plants and the best rhythms for activating them have only been carried out thanks to new methods and the collaboration of anthroposophical doctors.

I have used the names for the remedies as proposed by Rudolf Steiner solely in order to facilitate prescription and not as a means of disguised publicity.

Both Weleda (UK) Ltd., Heanor Road, Ilkeston, Derbyshire, DE7 8DR and Weleda, Inc. (www.weleda.co.uk) 175 North Ronte 9W, Congers, NY 10920, USA (www.usa.weleda.com) can supply full particulars of remedies not fully described in the text.

NOTES

Chapter 1
1. Steiner, R., *How to Knows Higher Worlds*, Anthroposophic Press, 1994.
2. Pfeiffer, E., *Sensitive Crystallization Processes. A Demonstration of Formative Forces in the Blood*, Anthroposophic Press, New York, 1975.
3. The expressions sympathy and antipathy will be used frequently and it is therefore necessary to state the specific meaning attributed to them here. The word sympathy sums up all that can impel one towards another being, and antipathy all that can repel. In short, all the movements of the soul can be related to one or other of these aspects in their widest sense.
4. For more on developing intuitive and clairvoyant faculties, see: Rudolf Steiner, *How To Know Higher Worlds*, Anthroposophic Press, 1994.
5. Carrel, A., and Lindbergh, C., *The Culture of Organs*, New York, Paul B. Hober, 1938.

Chapter 2
1. Steiner, R., *Spiritual Science and Medicine*, Rudolf Steiner Press, London, 1975.
2. Manterffel-Szoege, L., 'Remarks on Blood Flow', *Journal of Cardiovascular Surgery*, 10: 22–30. See also: Marinelli et al: 'The heart is not a pump', Frontier Perspectives, Fall–Winter 1995.

Chapter 3
1. See, for example, Steiner, R., *Occult Science—an Outline*, Rudolf Steiner Press, London, 1969.

Chapter 4
1. The expression 'separated' cannot exactly render an account of the reality, for it implies an idea of space that is inapplicable to

non-material elements. We can, nevertheless, for want of something better, use it if we are conscious that it only gives an *image* of the reality.

2. It may seem paradoxical to link the breaking down of tissue and structural organization. Nevertheless in the living world, the more developed an organ is as regards its form, the less vitality it possesses. Consider the nervous system, which is very complicated in structure but incapable of regeneration. Consider also the child, still very little formed but overflowing with vitality. Over-organization of structure leads to death just as a sculptor, searching for an ever more organized form, in carving and re-carving his statue, might leave nothing but a mass of scattered fragments.

3. Husemann, F., *Das Bild des Menschen als Grundlage der Heilkunst*, Verlag Freieis Geistesleben, Stuttgart, 1977.

4. Processes of inflammation and encystment can naturally also be methods of defence against a foreign body which has accidentally penetrated the organism and which will also remain impenetrable to its etheric forces.

5. With rare exceptions injections used in anthroposophical medicine are given subcutaneously. When the site of injection is not specified it should be made between the shoulders.

6. Potentization is a process of stepwise dilution, with shaking after each dilution. Starting with a plant extract, this is diluted to one in ten parts of water or grape sugar to give a 1x potency. One part of this dilution is diluted again in the same way, giving 2x, and so forth. Such potentized remedies are absorbed by the body without the need for a digestive process, giving a stronger and quicker effect. In general, low potencies 1–7 act on the metabolic system, intermediate ones 8–10 on the rhythmic system, and high potencies from 16 upwards on the nerve-sense system.

7. The 'vegetabilized' metals are obtained by growing suitable plants in soil enriched by the addition of a base of these metals. The plants grown in this manner are composted to serve the following year as an enrichment for a second generation of

plants. These in their turn serve as an enrichment for a third generation from which the remedy is extracted by the usual methods. We owe to Rudolf Steiner this method of 'dynamization' which raises the therapeutic properties of metals in a remarkable way and directs their action in accordance with the plant chosen.

8. Iron is present in small amounts throughout the body, and larger amounts in the red cells. Iron deficiency in human beings leads to weakness, loss of energy and will. One can deduce from this that iron promotes the integration of the ego and its will forces with the rest of the human being; in other words it promotes incarnation of the individuality.

Chapter 5

1. Steiner, R., *Spiritual Science and Medicine*, Rudolf Steiner Press, London, 1975. New edition: *Introducing Anthroposophical Medicine*, Anthroposophic Press, New York, 1999.
2. Husemann, F., *Das Bild des Menschen als Grundlage der Heilkunst*, op. cit.
3. See the *Meditations* series published by Rudolf Steiner Press, 2002.

Chapter 6

1. Healing by primary intention: where the edges of a wound progress to complete healing without scar formation or granulation.
2. Steiner, R., *Nine Lectures on Bees*, St George Publications, Spring Valley, 1964.

Chapter 7

1. Malson, L., *Les enfants sauvages, mythe et réalité*, Paris, 1964.
2. Glas, N., *Conception, Birth and Early Childhood*, Anthroposophic Press, New York, 1972.
3. Kesseler, E., 'Stillen und Brustkrebs', *Dtsch. med. Wschr.*, 93 (13), 1968.

4. zur Linden, W., *A Child is Born*, Rudolf Steiner Press, Sussex, 2004.
5. Glas, N., op. cit.
6. This is due to adequate sunshine during these months.
7. The same argument applies to measles vaccination. As described above, susceptibility to measles occurs as a result of difficulties in the incarnation process. Following an attack of measles children usually make sudden and marked strides in their development. Serious repercussions from whooping cough or measles are very rare in healthy children. If other illnesses are present then vaccination should be discussed as an option with an anthroposophical doctor. For more on the subject of vaccination, see the new, revised edition of: Goebels, W., and Glöckler, *A Guide to Child Health*, Floris Books, 2003.

Chapter 8
1. Cited by Husemann in *Das Bild des Menschen als Grundlage der Heilkunst*, p. 449, op. cit.

Chapter 10
1. Steiner, R., *The Four Temperaments*, Anthroposophic Press, New York, 1971.

Chapter 11
1. Schwenk, T., *Grundlage der Potenzforschung*, Schwäbisch-Gmünd, 1954.

Chapter 12
1. Steiner, R., *Introducing Anthroposophical Medicine*, op. cit.
2. This remedy, prepared by Wala Laboratories, is composed of *Cantharis* 4x/*Vesica urin.* 6x/*Equisetum* 3x/*Achillea* 3x for the granules, and 5x/6x/4x/4x respectively for the injections.

Chapter 13
1. For V. v. Weizsäckers, a throat inflammation is always the result of a situation of conflict that has not been overcome. A

total therapy must then (1) treat the throat inflammation, (2) balance the organism by moderating the exuberance of the metabolism and (3) help the patient to emerge from this situation of conflict.

2. This remedy, composed of *Primula/Onopordon/Hyoscyamus*, was the subject of a detailed study that appeared in *Correspondances Médicales* (Weleda, Saint Louis). We will therefore not consider it further in detail here, although we refer to it on several occasions. Briefly stated, it is a preparation that helps the heart to carry out its function of maintaining equilibrium and there are thus wide indications for its use.

3. Enos and Holmes, *J.A.M.A.*, 1953/XII, p. 1090.

4. R. Steiner.

5. We can see clearly that the control arising from the nerve-sense pole acts as a *brake* on the will. When this upper pole acts excessively, the will is so much restrained that it becomes paralysed. On the other hand, in the absence of control the will runs wild. Such a concept should encourage us to revise the idea of 'motor nerves', to which Rudolf Steiner was opposed.

Chapter 14

1. Holtzapfel, W., *Räumliche und zeithiche Ordnungen im Wachstum der malignen Tumoren*. Beiträge zu einer Erweiterung der Heilkunst, Stuttgart (1967/6).

2. Leroi, A., *Le cancer, maladie d'époque*, Triades, II/4, 1954. Leroi, A., *Causes et traitement du cancer*, Triades, XI/2, 1963. Leroi, A., *Le cancer, problème de la cellule ou de l'organisme?*, Triades, XIII/3, 1966.

3. Alexis Carrel: 'On the permanent life of tissues of the organism', in: *Journal of Experimental Medicine*, 1912.

4. Steiner, R., *Introducing, Anthroposophical Medicine*, op. cit.

5. Cohnheim, Julius; *Über Entzündung und Eiterung*, Leipzig 1914.

6. Leroi, A., *Cause et traitement du cancer*, op. cit.

7. Bauer, K. H., *Das Krebsproblem*, Berlin, 1949.

8. Bornfelt, J., *Arch. Hyg. Bakt.*, 249, 1960.

9. Kaelin, N., *Der Kapillar-dynamische Bluttest zur Frühdiagnose der Krebskrankheit*, Philosophisch-Anthroposophischer Verlag, Dornach, 1969.
10. Personal communication.
11. Since this book was written, a great deal of further research has been carried out. See for example: Kovacs, E.: 'The in vitro effect of *Viscum album* (VA) extract on DNA repair of peripheral blood mononuclear cells (PBMC) in cancer patients', *Phytotherapy Research 16*, 143–7: 2002. See also the *Report 2003* published by the Society for Cancer Research, Kirschweg 9, CH-4144 Arlesheim, Switzerland, e-mail: sekretariat@hiscia.ch
12. Blond, C., *The Liver and Cancer*, ed. John Wright, Bristol, 1960.
13. Pfeiffer, E., *Soil Fertility, Renewal and Preservation*, Faber and Faber, London, 1947.
    Kabisch, R., *Guide pratique de la méthode biodynamique*, Ed. Triades, Paris.

FURTHER READING

By Rudolf Steiner:

Extending Practical Medicine (with Ita Wegman), Rudolf Steiner Press, 1996

The Healing Process, Anthroposophic Press, 2000

Introducing Anthroposophical Medicine, Anthroposophic Press, 1999

An Introduction to Eurythmy, Rudolf Steiner Press, 1984

Medicine, An Introductory Reader (edited by A. Maendl), Rudolf Steiner Press, 2003

On general anthroposophy:

Anthroposophy in Everyday Life, Anthroposophic Press, 1995

The Effects of Esoteric Development, Anthroposophic Press, 1997

Harmony of the Creative Word, Rudolf Steiner Press, 2001

The Philosophy of Freedom, Rudolf Steiner Press, 1999

What is Anthroposophy?, Anthroposophic Press, 2002

Other authors:

Aeppli, Willi, *The Developing Child*, Anthroposophic Press, 2001

Cook, Wendy, *Foodwise*, Clairview Books, 2003

Hauschka, Rudolf, *Nutrition*, Rudolf Steiner Press, 2003

Hemleben, Johannes, *Rudolf Steiner, An Illustrated Biography*, Rudolf Steiner Press, 2000

Hydebrand, Caroline von, *Childhood*, Anthroposophic Press, 1988

Schwenk, Theodor, *Sensitive Chaos*, Rudolf Steiner Press, 1996

zur Linden, Wilhelm, MD, *A Child is Born*, Rudolf Steiner Press, 2004

INDEX

Abcesses, 64
Achillea millefolium, 50, 186
acne, 196
Aconitum, 55
Adonis vernalis, 146, 154
Agaricus muscarius, 195
ageing, 40, 61, 77, 100, 111, 139, 189
agoraphobia, 117
air organism, 15, 24, 94, 112, 113
albuminuria, 50, 131
alimentary tract, 19, 23, 24, 29–30, 35, 37, 44, 77, 121, 126, 130, 165
allergy, 111, 114–16
amenorrhoea, 183–5, 187
anabolic processes, 129–30
anaemia, 101, 102, 184
analgesics, 38
angina pectoris, 147, 148, 155
animals, animal kingdom, 10–16, 28, 63, 66, 71, 79, 96, 100, 132, 179, 189
antibiotics, 31, 65–6, 112
antibodies, 60
antimony, *see Stibium*
anuria, 131–2
Apis, 62, 64, 113, 139, 145, 153
Argentum, 44, 45, 51, 55–6, 65, 68, 135, 145, 153, 154, 185; *nitricum*, 136; *per Bryophyllum*, 44; *sulphuratum*, 56, 83
Arnica montana, 95–6, 148, 155, 198
arsenic, 93–4, 113, 131
Arsenic album, 113
arteriosclerosis, 56, 195
ascites, 119, 122
assimilation, 130, 134, 137, 139
asthma, 110–14, 116, 133, 190
astral (soul) body, 12–13, 15–17, 24–5, *and passim*; relation to air element, 12–13; relation to pain, 58
astral-ego complex, 17, 32
Aurum, 39, 54, 146, 148, 152, 153, 154, 155; *per Hypericum*, 146, 153; *per Primulam*, 148, 152, 154, 155
Avena sativa, 55

bacteria, 60, 65, 103–4, 144, 191
Belladonna, 55, 62–4, 113, 137, 145, 153, 154, 186, 197
Betonica, 97
Betula, 67, 193, 194–5
Bidor, 38–9, 52
bile, biliary complaints, 121–3, 124, 126
birch, 66–8, 95, 193, 194; *see also Betula*
Birch Elixir, 67–8, 195, 198
Blatta orientalis, 113
blood, 58, 60, 62, 129, 147, 151, 179; circulation, 21–3, 34, 140–1, 144, 147; red corpuscles, 140
Bolus eucalypti, 64, 84
bone, 81, 82, 162
bradycardia, 149
brain, 47
breast-feeding, 75–7, 133, 163
bronchitis (chronic), 112
Bryonia, 125, 145, 154
Bryophyllum, 43–4, 54
burns, 198

Cactus grandiflorum, 148, 154, 155
Calcarea carbonica, 110, 182, 183, 185
Calcium Supplements, 82–3, 97
calculi, 40, 123, 136; *see also* gallstones
Calendula, 194, 196–7
Camphora, 154
cancer, 51, 66, 89, 159–78; bladder, 166–7; breast, 75–6, 163, 169; liver, 168; pre-tumour period, 169–72, 178; prostate, 163; stomach, 168, 169; uterus, 163